Brain Agility

Peter Moulton, Ph.D.

Northwest Border Publications

Northwest Border Publications
P.O. Box 11752
Eugene, OR 97440 USA
info@nwbpub.com

ISBN 13:978-0-615-16166-2

Printed in the USA

Dedicated to everyone who is growing older.
As you age, may your mind remain youthful and gain wisdom.

Contents

Preface

This book is an outgrowth of an on-going interest as a psychologist in the rapidly developing abilities of neuroscience to investigate and influence the brain and of a desire to help older adults understand and deal with normal age-related cognitive decline. Brain imaging technology has dramatically increased our understanding of brain function. Neurofeedback technology now enables sophisticated monitoring of brain function and facilitates changes in brain behavior. Cognitive psychology now employs computer technology to exercise the brain, promoting enhanced cognitive functioning.

The realization that many individuals find paper and pencil more convenient and friendly than computers motivated the development of the Brain Agility Exercises, a program of paper and pencil exercises that can provide beneficial brain activity similar to that provided by computer exercises. A review of research and clinical studies shows that normal age-related cognitive decline can be forestalled and in many cases reversed by using paper and pencil exercises. Since most of these studies focus on only one or two areas of functioning, the findings of many studies were brought together in the development of the Brain Agility program. This program, based on current research, is designed to exercise and improve a wide range of cognitive functions including memory, attention, concentration, inductive reasoning, word fluency, visual-spatial orientation, and arithmetic skills. The 30 day Brain Agility program incorporates a uniform set of exercises with progressive levels of difficulty allowing initial success and providing increasing challenges as cognitive functioning improves.

Research in neuroscience, aging, psychology, and medicine shows the interdependence of the health of our bodies and our mental functioning. In light of this, it is important to place a program of mental exercise within the context of promoting a healthy lifestyle. Therefore, the first part of Brain Agility provides a basic understanding of brain function, its relationship to cognitive functioning, and how the brain is affected by nutrition, stress, and physical health. Guidelines are provided in each of these areas. An additional section discusses the complexity of memory and strategies for improving memory. A final section offers suggestions for resources for continued mental exercise.

Many people have contributed generously to the development of this book. In particular I would like to thank Marilyn Cohen, my wife, for her creative suggestions and valuable support. Several individuals, all accomplished writers, have reviewed the text and provided insightful comments and suggestions, greatly improving the book. I would especially like to thank Nancy Dahlberg, Craig Gilbert, Coral Mack, and Evon Smith. Finally, I would like to acknowledge the valuable comments and criticisms and the enthusiastic encouragement offered by the many participants in Brain Agility classes which have made use of the materials incorporated into this book.

It is my hope that everyone who reads this book and engages in the mental exercises will benefit and find growing older more enjoyable and rewarding.

Peter Moulton, Ph.D.
Eugene, Oregon
October 2007

Part I

The Agile Brain

Your Brain's Agility

An agile brain is quick, active, well organized, and has good recall. Brain Agility is about enhancing and maintaining your brain's ability to remember, stay focused, be aware and alert, and to enable you to enjoy life fully. This book describes how your brain functions, how it ages, and how to care for it. It is a "to do" book with a program of 30 days of mental exercises that can improve your cognitive functioning. These exercises are based on current research that shows how a program of exercises can increase blood flow to critical areas of your brain, stimulate the formation of new interconnections among areas of your brain, and promote more efficient brain function. Studies have demonstrated that mental exercise can also reduce the risk of developing brain diseases that may lead to dementia.

Your brain is the most important part of your body. It embodies the closest thing to "you." Your brain is the recipient of all of your senses and the repository of all of your memories. Without your brain no other part of your body would be able to function. Your brain's health determines your ability to think, to remember, to communicate, to perceive, to move about, and ultimately to live. It has been said that the body is the guesthouse of the mind. We could also say that the brain is the manager of the guesthouse. One of the most important ways of caring for yourself is caring for your brain.

As we age, we often find remembering faces and names more difficult. Words remain on the tip of our tongues and we increasingly have to make use of lists and other reminders. Senses become less keen and responses less quick. Vision and hearing -- the most important senses -- become less acute. We may have to ask a companion or spouse, "What did she say?" We may miss seeing a car entering the roadway. And the ability to slow our car or quickly change lanes may fail.

As these problems begin to occur, they create anxiety about cognitive decline. The major age-related concerns are loss of memory, impaired sensory functioning, fear of losing independence, and fear of disease resulting in dementia. It is important to distinguish between normal age-related decline and cognitive decline due to diseases of the brain. Fortunately, the cognitive decline most of us will experience is age-related. And, in most cases, the diminished memory and cognitive speed that we experience is offset by our knowledge, experience, and wisdom.

Clinical and longitudinal studies confirm that as our brains age our mental functioning declines.(refs.1,2,3) Memory begins to fail, word fluency declines, inductive reasoning becomes weaker, processing of sensory information becomes less discriminating, and our overall speed of processing slows. The steepest declines in mental functioning begin in the mid-sixties.

However, there is good news. One of the most important discoveries of neuroscience is that our brains can change and form new structures throughout our lifetimes. Much of age-related cognitive decline can be prevented. Where decline has occurred, some can be reversed and further decline forestalled, reducing the risk of developing dementia. Older adults are now maintaining independence longer.

The brain's ability to change and form new structures is called *brain plasticity*.(4,5) Not too many years ago common wisdom suggested age meant a loss of neurons in the brain and irreversible mental decline. We now know that the number of neurons in the adult brain declines very little and that some new neurons are actually formed. Much of age-related cognitive decline is due to a decrease of interconnections among neurons. However, *due to brain plasticity increased mental activity can form new interconnections.* In light of this, the dictum, "Use It or Lose It" has been commonly applied to the brain. A more positive dictum, forming the basis of Brain Agility, is "Use It and Improve It."

Numerous research studies have shown that mental stimulation maintains brain health and prevents cognitive decline. Increasing mental activity has also been found to reverse many cases of cognitive decline.(6,7,8) One of the most effective means of keeping your brain active is to engage in a program of mental exercise.

The recently expanded field of brain imaging, which can actually show the brain in action, dramatically reveals the ways in which mental activity promotes brain health. Functional Magnetic Resonance Imaging (fMRI) detects changes in the oxygen in blood as it is subjected to a magnetic field. The resulting images of the brain can show quite precisely those areas that are being used by particular cognitive functions such as memory, visualization, problem solving, and language.(9)

When we engage in mental activities drawing upon particular cognitive functions, blood flow increases to the corresponding areas of the brain. This can improve the health and function of those areas, increasing their capacity to serve the particular cognitive functions. Not only does the blood flow increase, but the development of new interconnections occurs among those areas.

For example, as we engage in an exercise involving the manipulation of visual images, we increase blood flow to the particular regions our brain uses for visual-spatial relations. These areas can then become healthier and develop new interconnections. This can then improve our ability to detect and process visual-spatial information in situations such as gauging the space between our car and other cars when parking.

Since different areas of our brain participate in different cognitive functions, a variety of mental exercises is important. The Brain Agility exercises have been specifically designed to activate a wide range of brain areas. Working on puzzles, such as crosswords or Sudoku, is beneficial. However, it is important not to limit yourself. Engaging in a variety of mental exercises, especially those where you may have less expertise, will activate areas of your brain that may have been getting less use.

In addition to mental activity, essential elements for maintaining brain agility are engaging in physical exercise, maintaining good nutrition, reducing stress, engaging in social activities, maintaining positive attitudes, and caring for any medical problems.(10)

To help understand why these elements are essential, the following chapters discuss brain basics and topics on how you can build and maintain an agile brain. Since a very important benefit of this book will come through the program of mental exercises, you may wish to begin the exercises in Part II as you continue with the following chapters.

Brain Basics

Brain Structure

The brain is truly amazing. It is the most complex organism of which we know. And we are constantly learning more about how it functions.

In size, our brains are relatively small, measuring about 6 inches by 5 inches by 5 inches and weighing about three pounds. About 75% of the brain is water. While the brain comprises only 2% of body weight, it consumes about 25% of our body's energy. The brain is the most protected organ. It is encased in a bone skull and floats in cerebrospinal fluid. The brain's blood supply (about 1.5 pints per minute) is protected by the blood brain barrier that prevents many potentially dangerous substances in the blood from passing into the brain. The brain also regulates its own blood pressure.

The brain's basic information processing unit is the neuron, the nerve cell that interacts with other neurons to receive and transmit information. There are approximately 100 billion neurons in an adult brain -- about 10% of all brain cells. Each neuron may interact with as many as 10,000 other neurons. Glial *glee-əl* cells, which comprise most of the remaining 90%, hold neurons in place, help supply nutrients and oxygen, insulate signals, destroy pathogens, and remove dead neurons.

Different types of glial cells provide particular supportive functions. Recent research is beginning to suggest that the glial cells may receive information from neurons and play a larger role in brain function. It was found that while the number of neurons in Albert Einstein's brain was not significantly different from normal brains, the number of glial cells in important areas was 40% greater than normal.(11)

The main components of a neuron are shown in Figure 1. The cell body contains the nucleus, mitochondria, and other components that maintain the life of the neuron. The dendrites receive signals from transmitting neurons. These signals may be propagated electrically through the axon and sent to other receiving neurons. As an electric signal is propagated, it is insulated by the myelin sheath that maintains efficient and reliable transmission. Signals are transmitted from axons to dendrites across a small gap called a synapse. This is a chemical process involving the transfer of neurotransmitters from the axons to the dendrites.

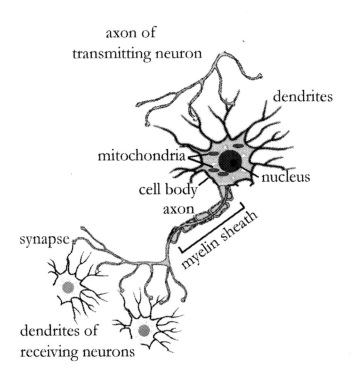

Figure 1. A Neuron

The human brain is organized into numerous areas and structures. The cortex is an outer layer of neurons about 2 millimeters thick, folded in order to fit its large surface area into the skull. Unfolded, it would be several square feet in size. The cortex enables thinking about and processing sensory inputs, emotions, memories, and other information that comes from the inner layers of the brain. It enables us to be uniquely human. The outside and inside structure of the brain is shown in Figure 2.

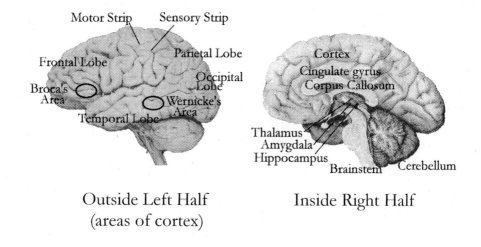

Outside Left Half
(areas of cortex)

Inside Right Half

Figure 2. The Brain

Particular cognitive functions are associated with corresponding areas of the cortex.

- *Frontal lobe* -- attention, processing emotions, planning, decision making, and problem solving.
- *Temporal lobe* -- auditory processing and language.
- *Occipital lobe* -- vision.
- *Parietal lobe* (containing the *sensory strip* and *motor strip)* -- processing sensory information about taste, touch, and movement, as well as controlling voluntary motor activities. It also is associated with reading and arithmetic.
- *Broca's area* and *Wernicke's area* -- language.

The cortex is divided laterally into the left hemisphere and right hemisphere. These are connected by the corpus callosum. The left hemisphere is faster and provides our logical reasoning, language and number abilities. The slower right hemisphere processes the gestalt or overall situation, leaving details to the left. It is associated with creativity and artistic abilities.

The limbic system, which lies under the cortex, is a more primitive brain structure that is common to most mammals. Some key structures within this are the hippocampus, which is the seat of memory, the amygdala which is the center of emotions, the cingulate gyrus, which is related to attention and emotional control, and the thalamus, which is a central switchboard within the brain.

It should be strongly emphasized that these descriptions provide only a very broad overview of the brain. There are many varied and detailed descriptions of brain areas and functions. Also, there are very complex interconnections between the various structures within the brain.

The Aging Brain

A human brain, especially the cortex, develops very rapidly following birth. It has the greatest number of neurons at age three. Childhood learning promotes increased interconnections among neurons and elimination of many unused neurons. By age 20, the number of interconnections among neurons reaches its peak.

A common misconception is that as we age, our neurons die off and cannot be replaced. More recent findings show that as we age we keep most of the neurons that we have at age 20. Also, recent evidence indicates that new neurons are spawned from stem cells in some areas of our brains. These stem cells can migrate to other areas producing new neurons. The discovery of neurotrophic factors that promote the growth of new neurons and new dendrites on existing neurons is an exciting new field of research. These discoveries promise the development of new methods of countering brain aging and brain disease.(12)

As we age, a number of physical changes occur resulting in cognitive decline:
- Blood flow decreases, reducing available oxygen and nutrients. Cardiovascular health determines blood flow throughout the body and especially the brain which consumes about 25% of the oxygen used by the body. Because this is so important, poor cardiovascular health is a strong predictor of cognitive decline.
- The density of dendrites decreases, resulting in fewer synaptic interconnections among neurons. As this happens, certain critical brain structures, such as the hippocampus which is central to memory, shrink. Also, the brain's normal ability to produce neurotransmitters is reduced, making them less available.

- Free radicals, which are generated by brain metabolism, damage cell walls and DNA of neurons and of mitochondria, small cell-like units within cells that convert food to energy. As they age, mitochondria become less efficient and produce a larger proportion of free radicals. At the same time, neurons are less able to neutralize the free radicals and thus become more vulnerable to their attack.

- As the brain becomes less efficient and suffers damage, spurious signals become more prevalent producing "noise."

The concept of "noise" can be illustrated by the images in Figure 3.

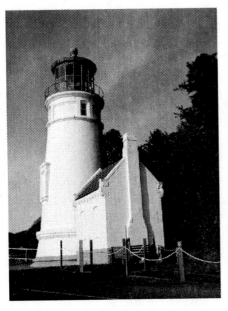

Lighthouse   "Noisy" Lighthouse

Figure 3. Noise

The image on the left is a normal photograph. The same photograph is on the right with noise introduced. To identify features in the image with noise requires more effort and time. When spurious signals arise in the brain and when other signals are inadvertently sent to the wrong neurons, it is as if noise has been introduced, requiring more effort and time for the brain to sort out the meaningful information.

As the brain ages, its processing speed declines. This is a common factor that underlies many of the cognitive deficits related to brain aging.(13,14) For

11

example, while we may not be able to recall the name of a person when we meet, given enough time, the name emerges. Similarly, although sorting out all of the things happening during a left turn at an intersection may be difficult, if the brain could work faster, the situation would be easily resolved.

Increase Your Brain Agility

The aging process can be moderated. While research has shown how the brain ages, it also has found that, regardless of age, brain plasticity provides some capacity to change and improve cognitive functioning. New interconnections between neurons can be formed and are formed throughout our lives. Mental exercise can develop new interconnections among neurons, increase supplies of neurotransmitters, and increase processing speed. Clinical studies have shown that mental exercise can stop and actually restore some losses in cognitive functioning. (15,16,17,18,19)

While plasticity offers the promise of new interconnections and changes in brain function, it does not guarantee that these changes will be for the better. As we age, we often become lazy and form "bad habits" of imprecise thinking. This is exemplified in imprecise use of language. We more frequently use pronouns rather than nouns and talk about "things" and "stuff." An important aspect of brain agility is maintaining precision and accuracy in language and all of our mental activity.

The most important key to brain agility is to stay mentally active. This means to stay active in a balanced way, not just keeping mentally busy. Balance should call upon a variety of cognitive functions and require dealing with new situations. Only in this way can you exercise the whole brain and promote growth that will maintain optimal cognitive functioning.

Staying mentally active should be fun and bring pleasure. Just as a healthy balance of physical activity should not cause on-going pain, a healthy balance of mental activity should not be something to be dreaded. Of course there may be some inertia to overcome at the beginning and new challenges may bring moments of embarrassment and anxiety. Keep in mind that what is important is to exercise, not to struggle, and not to base success on achievement.

Begin the Brain Agility Exercises

The Brain Agility 30-day program of exercises is the most unique part of this book. The program offers a valuable opportunity for you to exercise and improve your brain. The program is structured to allow scheduling 20 to 30 minutes of beneficial mental exercise each day. Since the exercises are so important, the entire second part of the book is devoted to them.

The exercises are balanced to challenge a broad range of cognitive functions. The variety and progressive difficulty are designed to maintain a productive challenge as your brain improves, to prevent boredom and keep you interested, and to provide some indication of your progress over the 30 days. If you have not already done so, you are encouraged to begin today.

Improve Attention

Most people think of the brain in terms of thinking, memory and problem solving. But the brain also controls attention, processes hearing, sight, and other senses, and coordinates critical motor functions such as balance. In many cases, normal age-related decline and deficits in a particular area can be prevented and improved by mental exercises that increase the brain's capacity to control and process these functions. One example of this is increasing attentional control.(20,21)

Attentional control is our ability to focus attention and to switch attention from one sensory stimulus to another. This is an essential brain function that underlies most of our daily activities. A much-studied instance of attentional control is dichotic listening, the ability to focus hearing in either the right or left ear.(22) Switching attention from one ear to another is required if we are attempting to talk with someone on a cell phone and alternately listen to the announcement in the airport. Another everyday instance of attentional control is our ability to quickly switch our attention from admiring the beautiful planter of flowers on the street corner to the child chasing a ball into the intersection.

As we age, our ability to rapidly switch and focus our attention declines. We find it more difficult to filter out background noise, and we may become more likely to have accidents. One very important prescription is to reduce the number of concurrent demands on our attention. A very good instance of this is to turn the cell phone off while driving! (23,24)

In addition to reducing distractions, the principle of brain plasticity and some research studies related to hearing and driving indicate that we can improve our attentional control. These and other studies have shown that hearing can be improved by exercising the brain. A simple exercise to improve hearing discrimination is to turn on a radio and the television at the same time, sit between them, and practice shifting your attention from one to the other. This will exercise both attentional control and the ability to filter out noise.

Other studies have shown that exercising our ability to visually attend to a wider field of vision can improve driving skills. Practice noticing how many items you can identify in a room or in an area outdoors. In addition, notice how many items you can identify in your peripheral vision while not moving your eyes.

Balance, a function of the brain, is another area in which age-related decline frequently occurs. Falling is one of the dangers and fears of growing old. Movement exercises such as tai chi and yoga have been found to increase balance and reduce the incidence of falling among the elderly. Even the simple exercise of standing on one foot (while holding on to a chair if necessary) will help improve balance.(25,26,27)

Learn Something New

Learning something new requires attention, concentration, remembering and working with new information, and some problem solving, all of which develop new synaptic connections. Many new activities also involve social interaction.

Some possibilities are:
- Learn a new language (or simply a few words and phrases such as common greetings), which develops auditory processing and memory. If you shop at an ethnic food store, you might learn to say "Hello", "How are you?", or "How much does this cost?" in the language of the shopkeeper.
- Learn a new skill such as painting, photography or playing a musical instrument. These activities will develop and strengthen areas of cognitive functioning such as visual processing, auditory processing, and auditory memory.
- Learn a new physical activity such as dancing or tai chi, which develops balance and physical health.

- Learn about a new subject such as a period of history, the life story of a famous person, or a scientific advance. This might be through attending a lecture or class, reading, using the internet, or using a set of CDs or DVDs.

Make Changes in Your Environment

Making changes in your environment takes you out of habitual routines. Although habits help us remember, they can also promote "brain laziness" and cognitive decline. Changes in your environment also make demands on attention, concentration, and memory. They make your environment richer which has been shown to improve cognitive functioning. Some possible changes are:

- Rearrange tools in your workshop, pots and dishes in your kitchen, or furniture in a room.
- Take a new route when traveling to work or to frequently visited shops. You will have to be more aware of where you are and what you are doing.
- Shop in a different supermarket or department store. You will have to search aisles and shelves and not depend on habit.
- Rearrange your schedule, perhaps changing meal times or when you watch news or other programs.

Engage in Social Activities

Social activity has been shown to be a very important factor in maintaining cognitive functioning as we age.(28,29) Social interaction requires auditory processing, language skills, attention, and memory. Even brief interactions can be of benefit. Some possibilities are:

- Ask a question or offer a comment. Ask store clerks if it has been a busy day, how long they have been working in that store, if they enjoy their work, or how they are able to remember the code numbers for all of the produce. Too often shoppers who spend the better part of an hour in a supermarket interact with others only to answer the questions, "Paper or plastic?" and "Debit or credit?"
- Join an organization. Book clubs, walking groups, garden clubs, political organizations, meditation, or yoga groups all offer varying

levels of social interaction in addition to their particular area of activity. Find one that meets your personal interests and needs. You might participate only occasionally or become a regular participant.

- Volunteer to help others (either a single event or an on-going commitment) such as helping an organization with mailings, assisting with registration at an event, or reading to others who cannot read. Helping others is the best method of feeling good.

What to Do?

With so many opportunities to increase your brain's agility, you might take a moment to consider how you might improve attention, learn something new, change your environment, or engage in more social activities. Make a few resolutions and write them in the space below.

Eat Wisely 4

Eating wisely provides our bodies and brains foods that are needed and avoids foods that can be harmful. The basic unit of our bodies and brains is the cell. Eating wisely supplies our bodies with the nutrients necessary to build and repair cells and above all provides energy for cells to live.

Free Radicals

The food we eat is converted to the life-energy necessary for cells by mitochondria contained within the cells. (See Figure 1) Mitochondria are organelles, similar to small cells within cells. They have their own DNA and can reproduce. The walls of mitochondria are made up primarily of fatty acids, and proteins. A neuron may contain a thousand or more mitochondria.

To provide energy to the cell for any bodily function, including neuron activity, mitochondria convert fats, proteins, and carbohydrates into complex molecules. This is a process requiring oxygen that we obtain by breathing.

While this process keeps cells alive, it also produces highly reactive forms of oxygen called free radicals.(30,31) The free radicals damage cells by combining with electrons from the fatty acids making up the mitochondria and cell walls. This process is called oxidation -- the same process that makes fats rancid. Oxidation damages the mitochondria and the cells. Free radicals can also damage the mitochondrial DNA.

This damage by free radicals reduces the efficiency of the mitochondria which causes them to produce a higher proportion of free radicals, escalating damage and inefficiency. Free radicals can also oxidize other lipids, polyunsaturated fats making up about half of the brain (excluding the water content). The damage by free radicals to the mitochondria and other important components of cells has been associated with cognitive decline and degenerative diseases such as Alzheimer's disease, cancer, diabetes, and cardiovascular disease. (32)

The brain produces more free radicals than any other organ. It is particularly vulnerable to free radical damage because of its large consumption of oxygen, its large content of polyunsaturated fats, and the fact that neurons do not divide (making repair of DNA damage difficult). Brains of victims of neurocognitive disease show changes consistent with free radical damage. Although cells produce enzymes that scavenge free radicals and repair damage, the battle is never ending, with age having the advantage. One current theory of aging attributes the aging process to the effects of free radicals.

Anti-Oxidants

Fortunately, many foods contain anti-oxidants that remove free radicals. Fruits and vegetables are particularly rich in anti-oxidants. The following table lists the most common anti-oxidants together with dietary sources. The information is taken from the National Institutes of Health Office of Dietary Supplements(33) and the United States Department of Agriculture(34):

Anti-Oxidant	Food Source (in order of potency)
Vitamin C:	citrus fruits, strawberries, cauliflower, spinach
Vitamin E:	wheat germ, almonds, sunflower seeds, spinach
Vitamin A:	carrots, spinach, vegetables, apricots, oatmeal
Niacin:	meat, fish, spinach, grains, nuts, mushrooms (deficiency related to risk of Alzheimer's disease)
Vitamin B-6:	baked potato, banana, chicken, oatmeal
Folic Acid:	fortified cereals, dried beans, leafy vegetables (folic acid masks B-12 deficiency, combine with B-12 to avoid neural damage)
Vitamin B-12:	clams, fortified cereal, fish, beef (important for neural repair)
Flavanoids:	tea, coffee, soy, chocolate, red wine
Lycopene:	tomatoes, watermelon, pink or red grapefruit
Selenium:	Brazil nuts, tuna, beef, egg, cottage cheese

All of these anti-oxidants are also available as dietary supplements.

Dr. Martha Morris, of the Rush Institute for Healthy Aging, led a study of 815 Chicago residents between 1993 and 2003 that found that those with the highest levels of dietary vitamin E (highest fifth) had a risk of Alzheimer's disease 67% lower than those with the lowest vitamin E consumption. No significant change in risk was found for those taking only vitamin E supplements, other antioxidants, or a general vitamin.(35)

Dr. Morris and her team also found that those with higher levels of dietary Niacin intake had less incidence of Alzheimer's disease and experienced slower rates of cognitive decline. Other studies indicate that the benefit of Niacin in preventing Alzheimer's disease does not occur if there is a deficiency of vitamin B-12.(36)

A study in the Netherlands examined 5395 participants aged 55 and over in 1990-1993, 1993-1994 and 1997-1999. All of the participants were free of dementia and non-institutionalized at the beginning of the study. Six years later 197 participants developed dementia of which 146 had Alzheimer's disease. High intake of vitamin C and vitamin E were associated with a significantly lower risk of Alzheimer's disease. This was especially true for smokers who also benefited from intake of beta carotene, a form of vitamin A, and flavanoids.(37)

Dr. Jane Durga, of Wageningen University in the Netherlands, led a study of 818 participants aged 50 to 70 that found that individuals given 800 micrograms of folic acid daily experienced less cognitive decline after three years. They were found to be 4.7 years younger in overall memory functioning and 6.9 years younger in delayed recall memory.(38)

One particularly strong anti-oxidant that deserves attention is curcumin which is found in turmeric, a common Indian spice. Curcumin is not only a strong antioxidant but is an effective anti-inflammatory and anti-fungal. It has been called the "Asian Aspirin." In addition, laboratory studies have found that curcumin prevents and removes amyloid plaques from the brain.(39) These are associated with Alzheimer's disease. This may in part explain the very low prevalence of Alzheimer's disease in India where turmeric is used in many foods. About 3% of Americans between the ages of 70 and 79 suffer from Alzheimer's. The number in India is about 0.7%. Clinical studies are underway in the U.S. to investigate this property of curcumin. Turmeric has a concentration of curcumin of about 4%. Curcumin is also available as a dietary supplement. While there is no established recommended dietary allowance of turmeric, there is no known toxic level. Some clinical studies have administered up to 12 grams of curcumin per day. Many sources recommend three grams per day or about one and a half teaspoons of turmeric. An excellent review of curcumin is provided by the Linus Pauling Institute at Oregon State University.(40)

Acetyl-l-carnitine , often called Alcar, is a compound that has been shown to increase mitochondrial efficiency in producing energy in cells. Laboratory and clinical studies of Alcar have shown that it improves both physical and brain functioning. However, this greater mitochondrial efficiency comes with the cost of a higher production of free radicals. To counter this, acetyl-l carnitine has been combined with Alpha-lipoic acid, a strong anti-oxidant.(41)

Fats

Fats play a critical role in brain nutrition. About 70% of the brain is water, and over half of the remainder is made of fats. These are in the form of polyunsaturated fats that are particularly vulnerable to damage by oxidation. The brain needs fats to build cells and repair cell structures.

There are two important issues in dealing with dietary fats. First, hydrogenated and trans-polyunsaturated fats are to be avoided. Second, sufficient polyunsaturated fats are needed.(42,43)

Hydrogenated fats, which include trans-fats, are fats that have been combined with hydrogen by industrial processes. This produces a fat that resists becoming rancid and hence has a longer shelf life. For this reason these fats are used in many processed foods. However, hydrogenated fats can bind to cell walls and interfere with normal metabolic processes. This can lead to cell starvation, toxicity and cell death.

At Rush Institute for Healthy Aging, 815 community residents aged 65 and older unaffected by Alzheimer's disease were studied over an average of 3.9 years. The 20% of the group with the highest intake of saturated and trans-fats had 2.2 times greater risk of Alzheimer's disease than the 20% with the lowest intake. Total fat, animal fat, and dietary cholesterol were not associated with Alzheimer's disease.(44)

Dietary polyunsaturated fats do not present this danger. These include the omega-3 fatty acids that are especially important for brain health: linolenic acid

(LNA), linoleic acid (LA), eicospentaenoic acid (EPA), and docosahexaenoic acid (DHA). Flax seed, soybean, canola, wheat germ and walnuts are sources of LA and LNA. Although the body can produce some EPA and DHA from LA and LNA, the major sources of EPA and DHA are fish.

The Framingham Heart Study examined 899 men and women over a 9 year period. The average age at the beginning of the study was 76 years. At the end of the study 99 new cases of dementia occurred. Those who ate three servings of fish per week had a significant 47% reduction in the risk of developing dementia.(45)

General Dietary Guidelines

This section has focused on the role good nutrition plays in maintaining optimal brain health. Since any health problems in other parts of your body can directly or indirectly affect your cognitive functioning, providing good nutrition for your whole body is equally important. The recent nutritional guidelines established by the U.S. government recommend eating daily: (46)

- 5 to 10 ounces of grains (this might be one slice of bread -- preferably whole grain, a half-cup of cooked rice or pasta, or a cup of ready-to-eat cereal);
- 2 to 3 $1/2$ cups of a variety of vegetables;
- 1 $1/2$ to 2 $1/2$ cups of fruit;
- 3 cups of milk products (1 cup of milk equals $1^1/_2$ to 2 ounces of cheese or 1 cup cottage cheese);
- 5 to 7 ounces of meat poultry, fish, or the equivalent (1 egg, $1/_4$ cup of cooked beans or tofu, $1/_2$ ounce of nuts or seeds, or 1 tablespoon of peanut butter are equivalent to 1 ounce of meat).

These recommendations are very general and will vary according to your level of activity and any food restrictions due to allergies and food intolerances. You are encouraged to read some of the many materials that are available through governmental agencies and organizations dedicated to healthy aging. (47) Minimum daily requirements of nutrients and recommended dosages of supplements can be obtained from these sources and should be discussed with your health care provider.

What to Do?

This might be a good time to review what nutritional changes you can make to improve your brain health and to write them in the space below.

Maintain Physical Fitness 5

Maintaining physical fitness throughout your life is one of the best keys to preventing cognitive decline. One study showed that dementia in later life could be predicted 20 years in advance by the presence of hypertension, hypercholesterolemia, and obesity, as well as age and education.(48)

Research has shown that individuals with high cardiovascular fitness as well as those who undergo six months of aerobic training have increased activity in areas of the brain associated with attentional networks, spatial selection, and inhibitory functioning. Aerobic training increases cortical capillary supplies, development of interconnections between neurons, and the growth of neurons.(49)

A study of 4615 Canadians aged 65 and older found that those with high levels of physical activity were half as likely to develop cognitive impairment or Alzheimer's disease.(50) A study of 2288 adults 65 and older in Seattle indicated that the incidence rate for dementia for the high activity group was one-third of that for the low activity group.(51) Physical activity can include performance-based tasks such as raking leaves or sweeping a floor.

If your cardiovascular system is not functioning well, one of the best things you can do for your brain is to improve your cardiovascular health. This may involve seeking medical care for any cardiovascular problems, changing diet, getting more physical exercise, and reducing stress. If your cardiovascular health is good, one of the most important ways to prevent cognitive decline is to maintain its good health.

In addition to maintaining cardiovascular health, other chronic conditions such as diabetes, obesity, and thyroid dysfunction have been shown to significantly contribute to cognitive decline. For the sake of your brain, it is important to maintain the highest level of physical health possible.

Physical exercise is one of the most beneficial elements of any healthy lifestyle. There are four categories of physical exercise, all of which are important for the health of your brain:

- Aerobic or endurance exercise such as brisk walking
- Strength or resistance exercise such as lifting a weight
- Stretching exercise such as bending to touch your toes
- Balance exercise such as standing on one foot

Aerobic exercise improves cardiovascular health by increasing heart rate and breathing. For an older fit person, 15 to 20 minutes of brisk walking three times a week has been shown to decrease the risk of cognitive decline. A rule of thumb for such exercise is that if you can talk without difficulty while exercising, you should exert more effort; and if you cannot talk at all, you are exerting too much effort. Other forms of aerobic exercise are climbing stairs and, especially for those with joint problems, swimming.

Strength or resistance exercise requires that you exert effort against some force, most often gravity. This of course develops muscular strength. A simple beginning exercise might be simply lifting your arms from the side of your legs to above your head, or lifting your forearms to your shoulders. This might be repeated 10 or 20 times. As strength is developed, weights can be added such as holding a can of food in each hand.

Stretching exercises develop flexibility in the body. When combined with the other exercises, stretching has been shown to increase the benefit of the other exercises in preventing cognitive decline. Stretching might be as simple as reaching for the ceiling or the floor or as precise as a yoga posture.

Balance exercises are very important for the elderly. In addition to improving brain health, they help prevent falls, which in the worse case can result in inactivity that then reduces brain health.

Following are basic guidelines for any exercise program:

- If you have any physical problems, consult with your health care provider before beginning.
- Start slowly and build up.
- Take time to warm up at the beginning of each exercise session.

- Although some muscle soreness might be experienced at the beginning, exercise shouldn't be painful.
- Take time to cool down at the end of the exercise session.

Starting and maintaining an exercise program requires discipline and encouragement.

Following are some guidelines for a walking program:
- Set a schedule, perhaps a 15 to 30 minute session three times a week.
- Even if you feel that you might not be able to complete the session or don't want to exercise, show up. (As Woody Allen said, "Eighty percent of success is showing up on time.").
- Make a commitment with a friend (social commitment is a strong motivator).
- Get a pedometer, which counts the number of steps taken, to measure your progress in each session.
- Keep track of your progress and compliment yourself on your success.

The purpose of this section is not to present a physical exercise program, but to indicate the importance of physical exercise and to outline some major guidelines. There are many excellent resources for exercise programs, some of which are included in the further reading section at the end of the book.

What to Do?

You are encouraged to take a few minutes to review the amount and type of your exercise during a typical week. Do you get aerobic exercise for 15 to 30 minutes three to five times a week? Could you benefit from strengthening or stretching exercises? How is your balance? In the space below and on the next page you might write some of the ways in which you could improve your brain health through exercise.

Relax Your Body and Brain 6

Stress is produced by any change that requires adaptation. The change may be perceived as good or bad. Stress may result from life events: marriage or divorce, promotion or demotion, birth of a child or death of someone dear. Stress may be caused by challenging physical circumstances, even the weather. Chemicals such as air pollution can cause stress. Our thoughts can also be stressful: excitement, fears, worries, exuberance, and remorse.

Stress mobilizes the body by increasing blood pressure, heart rate, and glucose levels as well as by producing hormonal changes. Mentally, stress raises our level of arousal, which can facilitate heightened attention and mental functioning. If we are threatened, this mobilization prepares us for dealing with the threat: the "fight or flight response." If the stressors are perceived as desirable, such as a promotion, we are ready to celebrate.

If we are in a situation where either fighting or running is appropriate, stress has prepared us for action. In this case the stress is adaptive and can be considered "good." However, when there is nothing we can do about the situation, the activation of our body and mind without any subsequent release of this energy can be harmful. If the stressors are recurrent, such as in an aversive work setting, chronic stress can lead to burnout, physical disease, cognitive decline, and depression.

To understand how stress works, it is useful to understand how the brain interacts with the adrenal glands. This is a complex process involving two pathways illustrated in Figure 4. The Hypothalamus-Pituitary-Adrenal Cycle involves the brain sending hormones to the adrenals that in turn send hormones back to the brain. The other pathway involves direct neural stimulation of the adrenal glands.

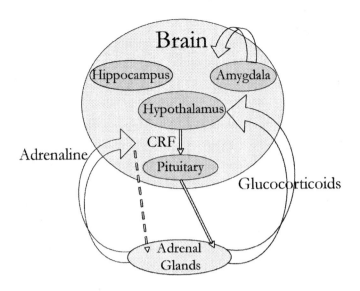

Figure 4. Hypothalamus-Pituitary-Adrenal Cycle

When your brain perceives a stressor, the hypothalamus, part of the limbic system, releases corticotrophin releasing factor (CRF). CRF activates the pituitary gland that then produces adrenocorticotrophic hormone (ACTH). ACTH travels in the bloodstream to the adrenal glands where it activates the production of glucocorticoids and other hormones. One important function of these hormones is to increase energy reserves in the body by converting protein and lipids to carbohydrates. Cortisol, one of these hormones, travels through the bloodstream back to the hypothalamus where it moderates the production of CRF. The brain also sends nerve signals to the adrenal glands causing them to produce epinephrine and norepinephrine. These two hormones help prepare for fight or flight.

While the production of the many hormones related to stress can facilitate meeting challenges, glucocorticoids can also adversely affect memory and learning. Experiments in which subjects were given tablets containing cortisol over a four day period showed disruption of verbal memory.(52) Fortunately this reversed when the cortisol was no longer administered. Cortisol can block glucose utilization by brain cells which can have an immediate effect on memory. Long term exposure to high levels of cortisol correlates with increased hippocampal shrinkage in normal elderly adults. This shrinkage results in decreased memory.(53) Chronic stress can also promote many diseases, such as diabetes, arthritis, cancer, heart disease, hypothyroidism, and osteoporosis. In turn, diseases such as diabetes, heart disease, and hypothyroidism can also adversely affect brain function.

Reducing Stress

The first step in reducing stress is to identify the stressors provoking the stress. Too often stressors are seen as part of life and are not dealt with consciously. One method of recognizing stressors is to note when you feel exhausted, frustrated, angry, fearful, worried, or over-excited. Ask yourself what is happening, especially if there is something you wish were otherwise but feel you can't control. Make a list, especially of events that occur frequently.

External stressors such as extremes of heat or cold, environmental pollution, or sleep deprivation can often be dealt with through environmental and life style changes. Internal stressors are usually emotional responses such as fear, anger, worry, and over-excitement. While these too can sometimes be dealt with by external changes, they often require changes in attitude and learning to moderate emotional responses.

Many of the stressors in our lives are part of the unnecessary clutter we have accumulated. Simplifying can make life less stressful. There is a Tibetan saying, "If you have a pound of tea, you have problems the size of a pound of tea. If you have a horse, you have problems the size of a horse." This is not to suggest giving away all of your belongings. However, do consider letting go of any object, interpersonal relationship, or habit that creates stress and offers little benefit. If watching the news usually leaves you upset, limit the time you watch it. If caring for houseplants becomes an unpleasant and often put-off chore, consider reducing the number you have.

Routines may also be part of unnecessary clutter. If you feel burdened by having to prepare a three course meal at dinner time, find some simple one-pot meals, perhaps ones you can prepare in advance. Your family will likely appreciate less stress in the air. Disorganization can also be a form of stressful clutter. Searching unsuccessfully for a misplaced receipt or document can be very stressful. Organizing papers you have to keep and discarding those you don't have to keep will reduce both your clutter and your stress.

Worrying is one of the stressors most of us can do without. Worry is usually fear of some future event. Having some sense of control over the situation can reduce the worry. An example might be an upcoming doctor's appointment. If you know of or suspect a particular illness, learn more about it to become better informed. You might create a list of specific health concerns and questions to ask and document specific symptoms and frequency of their occurrence. Then you might discuss these with someone who can go to the appointment with you to help remember to ask all of the questions and to help write down the information and instructions given by the doctor. Planning a course of action will help quell the stressful cycling of worry.

If you really cannot do much to change a situation, try to view it as positively as possible. Dwelling on how bad a situation is will only make it more stressful. Some things in life cannot be changed. Try to focus on areas of your life where you do have control.

In general, maintaining a positive attitude reduces your stress. Have a sense of humor about things that don't go exactly according to plan. Develop flexibility and the ability to change course rather than fighting the storm.

Relaxation is a universal tool for reducing stress. Learning to relax can significantly benefit both your body and mind and will promote brain health. The simplest relaxation technique is to take a deep breath. When stressed we tend to tighten our muscles and not breathe freely. Studies have shown that taking a deep breath immediately reduces our heart rate.

Another very simple relaxation technique is to look about, name five items that you see, and note their color. This technique can be done with any of your senses. You can take note of sounds about you or note the feel of your feet on the floor, your seat in the chair or the position of your shoulders and hands. Focusing on immediate sensations shuts off busy and stressful thoughts. This momentarily reduces stress allowing a break that may provide an opening to change your situation.

Yoga, Tai Chi, and Qi Gong are other well known practices that promote relaxation, physical health, and well being. Since the 1970s a number of formal eastern meditation techniques have become popular in the West. Many research studies show that meditation calms the mind and body and can reduce stress. The following outlines the basic steps for a meditation practice that will produce a calm state of mind.

Breathing Meditation Technique

To use the breath as the focus of meditation:

1) Find a quiet room free of distractions. While this is important at the beginning, your ultimate goal is to be able to relax in stressful situations that are generally not quiet. Some meditators find practicing in a crowded bus station is beneficial.

2) Sit comfortably with your back straight. This can be in a chair or on a cushion with your legs crossed.

3) Gently place your attention on your breath, allowing it to be natural. Do not try to make it slow or regular or light.

4) Leave your eyes open if possible. While closing your eyes shuts off visual distractions, closing off other senses is more difficult. Just as you can meditate with other senses open, you can meditate with your eyes open. When you bring the relaxation of meditation into a stressful situation you will usually need to have your eyes open. Also, opening your eyes will usually keep you more alert and less sleepy.

5) Thoughts will come to mind. As they do, try to be aware of their presence and do not get carried away on a train of thought. When you realize that your attention has drifted away from your breath, gently bring it back.

6) If you find holding your attention on your breath difficult, you might count the number of exhalations, counting 7 or 21 and then repeat the count.

7) Do this for a few minutes and then allow yourself to focus on other features of your surroundings. Without getting up, move your head, arms, and shoulders if they have become stiff or uncomfortable.

8) After a few moments, return your attention to your breath as in steps (3)-(6).

9) Repeat this process three or four times for a total of 15 to 20 minutes. If time seems to go very slowly, shorten the sessions. If time seems to go very quickly you might lengthen the sessions.

What to Do?

Before continuing to the next section you might think about the stressors in your life and in the space below make a list of the most prominent ones. Then consider and write out ways in which you might deal with these so that they might have less impact on your life and your brain.

Remember to Remember

Memory is one of the most basic brain functions. Our memory tells us what we have done, whom we have known, and where we have been. It holds all that we have learned. We have many different memories: past experiences, the name of an acquaintance, the telephone number we've just seen in the directory, and how to make a cup of tea.

Poor memory is the most common age-related cognitive complaint. We find that our nouns get lost and we resort to talking about "her" or "they" or "things." We may forget to water the plants and may have trouble recalling the day of the week. These failings bring up fears of losing completely one's memory and mind. About 30% of normal, healthy adults over age 50 have concerns about poor memory.(54) Just as our bodies become less agile with age, our brains, which are part of our bodies, become less agile. However, it is important to realize that in spite of not being able to remember a name or a date you retain many memories. You probably remember whether or not you like chocolate! Also, there are ways to improve memory. To understand these it is useful to examine the nature of memory.(55)

Memories come in different modalities. There are memories of sensory experiences. We may remember the beauty of a rose, its fragrance, the prick of a thorn, or the sound of the hummingbird feeding from the flower. There are memories of emotions: we may remember the joy when first seeing the rose and the sadness at seeing it wither. Many memories are factual. These may be remembered as verbal statements.

Those areas of the brain that were activated in the original experience are reactivated when we remember the experience. When you recall eating a sour dill pickle, your brain goes through the process of tasting, seeing, and smelling much in the same way that it did with the actual pickle. You may even find saliva flowing! Also, memories are reworked each time we remember them. Feelings, judgments, and new associations may be added.

Emotions can play an important role in memory. An experience associated with a strong emotion is more likely to be remembered. The emotion itself is often the key to retrieving the memory.

Phases of Memory

Establishing and recalling memory entails three phases: input, storage, and retrieval. The input phase acquires information through sensory and cognitive processes. When meeting new people, we see their faces and hear their names. This input information is then consolidated and stored. At some later time we see their faces again and retrieve the information, remembering meeting them and hopefully remembering their names.

Not being able to remember can be due to difficulties with any of these phases. In order to acquire information we have to pay attention. Distraction by competing stimuli such as fatigue, pain, or anxiety may interfere with attention and cause some information to be lost. Often our thoughts, such as thinking about our response to what is happening, become the distraction. Sensory failure due to poor eyesight, hearing loss, noise, weak sounds, or dim lighting can reduce the amount and quality of the information acquired.

In order to store information we must have some way of organizing or indexing the information. To do this we develop semantic maps that link associated items of information. If an experience is entirely novel and without precedent, our brains may have difficulty finding the place to store the information. This is the case when listening to something new. Lack of sleep, medications, and other substances that affect brain function can also result in poor consolidation and storage.

Retrieval of information requires a key into our semantic map -- a piece of information that links to the information we want. If we cannot find the key, we cannot access the information in spite of its sitting there in our memory. We haven't forgotten; we just don't know how to reach it. The process of finding our way into the semantic map explains why we "warm up" to a subject and recall more and more information as we talk or think about it.

Types of Memory

There are many schemes for categorizing aspects of memory. Temporally we can speak of *short term* memory and *long term* memory. The telephone number of the local bookstore is something we need remember for the 15 to 30 seconds from finding it in the telephone directory until dialing it. To remember this number for the rest of the month would only be burdensome. However, we would like to remember our own telephone number for as long as we have it.

Working memory is a special form of short term memory. It holds information in our currently active memory while we manipulate it. A common test of short term memory is to repeat a string of digits backwards. We must hold the original string in our working memory while reversing the digits. An everyday example of working memory is to determine at what time you must leave home in order to complete a number of errands before your 4:00 pm doctor's appointment. Perhaps you need 15 minutes to reach the post office, 10 minutes to mail a package, 20 minutes to drive to the hardware store, 15 minutes to select and purchase the paint for the bookcase, 10 minutes to drive to the cleaners and pick up your clothing, and 15 minutes to drive to the doctor's office. Thus, after some manipulation of this information in your working memory, you determine that you need 85 minutes for the errands and must leave home at 2:30 pm to give yourself 5 minutes leeway.

If your mind becomes boggled when you have to mentally manipulate a schedule of times such as this, you can assume that the capacity of your working memory is being exceeded. Normally we can hold five to nine items in our working memory. Beyond that we have to use paper and pencil.

Long term memory contains our history and the information we have learned over time. It can be divided into *explicit* and *procedural* memory. Explicit memory holds information about events and facts. Many of our daily routines are stored in procedural memory.

Long term memory can be further divided into several functional categories.
- *Episodic memory* holds information about events such as what you ate for dinner last night and where you spent last New Year's Eve.
- *Knowledge* is learned information such as how sunlight and raindrops produce rainbows.
- *Source memory* holds information about the source of information such as your having read about the price of oil in yesterday's newspaper.
- *Prospective memory* remembers that you have to do something such as mail a letter or turn off the water before the tub overflows.

- *Personal memory* holds information about yourself such as your enjoying spending time with a particular person.
- *Procedural memory* holds information about how to do something such as making a cup of tea or pruning an apple tree.

Memory and the Brain

There is no one memory center in the brain. The hippocampus plays a major role in long term memory. However, the cerebellum and basal ganglia hold procedural memory. This explains why some people may have great difficulty recalling past events but retain the ability to learn and follow routines. These memory areas are linked to many other brain areas. While the hippocampus tends to hold detailed information related to specific experiences, the cortex holds more generalized or consolidated information. The consolidated information is sometimes referred to as semantic memory.

As the human brain ages, the hippocampus shrinks at the rate of about 2% per decade beginning around age 40.(56) Certain diseases accelerate this rate. In addition, neurotransmitter production diminishes, slowing brain function. Receptors important to memory also diminish in number.

Normal, healthy aging brings memory lapses to all but a very few. The good news is that these do not signal the onset of a dementia and that there are many strategies that will improve memory.

Improving Memory

The most important rule for good memory is to pay attention. Thinking of something else while listening to someone or while reading a book ensures you will miss what was said or read. Being distracted by irrelevant sights and sounds prevents acquiring the information to be remembered. Even being over-anxious about not remembering can be a distraction. It is important to relax.

When meeting new people, look at them. If necessary, ask them to repeat their name. If the name is unusual, ask how to spell it. Note facial features, tone of voice, posture, and dress. Every item of information can provide a linkage for storing and retrieving information. If the setting in which you are meeting a person is distracting, try to move to a quieter place.

When reading, turn off the television. Don't try to read something important when also listening for the pot to boil or the dog to scratch at the door. Strong emotions or excitement about an event unrelated to what is being read or listened to are likely to be significant distractions. It may be best to calm down first.

Once information has been acquired, using it will help consolidate it, making retrieval easier. When hearing someone's name, repeat it -- aloud if possible. Tell someone else about the person you met, including their name. When creating a shopping list or to-do list, repeat it aloud -- perhaps several times. After reading an article, summarize it to yourself or someone else. Ask yourself why the information is important.

Forming associations between new information and what is already known helps the brain make linkages in semantic memory. Pay attention to the place where you meet a new person. Identifying a distinctive feature of the person will facilitate making associations. Identify common acquaintances, common interests, and common history. When reading or watching a television program you wish to remember, ask yourself how the new information might change what you already know. Ask why it is important. Will you want to act on it in some way?

Forming associations can also help you remember to do something. Perhaps when going to bed you might remember that you forgot to water the plants. You might then tell yourself that you will remember when you start to drink your first cup of coffee the next morning. Visualize yourself doing this and repeat the instruction -- aloud if possible.

As mentioned above, memories gain strength if they are associated with emotions. Noting and feeling the emotion that an experience or information evokes can help store and retrieve a memory.

To remember a list, cluster information so that several items can be handled as a single item. This is commonly done with telephone numbers. Rather than having to remember the 10 digits 5416889041, we remember the area code (541), the prefix 688, and the number 9041. This technique can be used with many lists. The items of a shopping list might be clustered according to meat, dairy, and produce.

One of the best methods to improve prospective memory is to create routines. This shifts the memory from prospective memory to procedural memory which is much more robust. You might develop a routine to take medications immediately after breakfast, after the morning news, or in relation to some other daily activity.

In addition to the internal methods just discussed, there are several external memory aids. The most common is to create a written list such as a shopping list or to-do list. Carrying a small notebook in which to write notes and things to do or buy can be an important memory support.

Organizational aids such as calendars can reinforce prospective memory. Timers as well as alarm clocks remind us what to do. Another aid for prospective memory is to place an item in an unusual and prominent location. Before going to bed you might place a toothpaste tube on the breakfast table as a reminder of a dental appointment the next day. Placing the telephone on the floor can be a reminder to phone to have the car tuned up. Finally, asking someone to remind you may work best, especially if the other person enjoys helping you or conversely reminding you of what you've forgotten.

There are many good resources for more information on memory and memory strategies. Some are listed in the references (55) and the section on further reading.

Part II

The 30-Day Program
of
Brain Agility Exercises

The Brain Agility Exercises are designed to help adults maintain cognitive functioning and in many cases to help recover losses due to age-related cognitive decline. They are based upon current research that has shown the importance and value of mental exercise. While they may be of benefit in cases involving medical conditions, the exercises are not designed as cures for medical conditions that affect cognitive functioning and are offered as education and not in lieu of medical treatment. If you are experiencing cognitive decline due to a medical condition, it is important to seek medical advice and treatment.

Overview of the Exercises 8

The Brain Agility exercises are designed for about 20 to 30 minutes of daily mental exercise. In addition to daily memory and naming exercises, there are nine other categories of exercises that challenge visual, verbal, numerical, and logical functioning. For variety, only six of the nine are presented for a given day. The different types of exercises call upon corresponding cognitive functions in order to stimulate the brain structures underlying these functions. The variety also gives freshness to your daily mental exercise. In the following sections an introductory description of each category is given together with suggestions for strategies. Of course there is no one best strategy and you may find your own methods for solving the problems.

Most exercises have blanks where you can record the time you spend on the exercise. Working quickly to improve mental processing speed adds considerable benefit to the exercises. If you have or can obtain a timer, do record your times. This will also provide an approximate indication of progress. However, many exercises become more difficult as the days progress and may require more time. Doing your exercises at the same time each day will also allow a more accurate comparison of performance. Most people are at their highest levels of mental performance in the morning.

Some exercises may seem very easy and others quite challenging. The different types of exercises will stimulate different parts of your brain. It is important to keep in mind that the exercise is more important than the struggle! The exercise will stimulate blood flow to your brain, keep your neurons active, and build new interconnections. If a particular exercise seems extremely difficult, don't get stuck; move on to the next without feeling badly. You will get good exercise whether you win the race or come in last. However, do not become too lax. While doing the best that you can as quickly as possible, the real measure of success is how much you gain over a month of exercising. As you develop your "mental muscles," you will not only feel good about doing so but will find that your brain is functioning better in the course of everyday living.

The solutions to the exercises are given beginning on page 249.

There are 30 days of exercises -- enough for a month. However, if you miss a day, don't worry. Do only one set of exercises a day and try to finish within six weeks. And enjoy your healthier, happier brain!

Sequences

A Sequence exercise presents five elements of a sequence and challenges you to find the next element. This exercises your short term and working memory, your abilities to recognize similarities and differences among the elements and your abilities to form and test hypotheses. All of these are important in everyday problem solving.

In many cases the sequences will rely upon well-learned sequences such as the alphabet and numbers. In other cases numbers and letters are used as symbols without regard to numeric or alphabetic order. In general the key to the solution is to examine the relationship among differences between successive pairs of elements in the sequence.

For example, given the sequence:

$$1 \quad 3 \quad 5 \quad 7 \quad 9 \quad \underline{\hspace{1cm}}$$

You can easily determine that the difference between each pair is 2 and that the next element should be 11.

Given the sequence:

$$2 \quad 3 \quad 5 \quad 9 \quad 17 \quad \underline{\hspace{1cm}}$$

the differences between successive pairs are 1, 2, 4, 8. Here the differences are not constant, but are doubled at each step. The differences themselves are an increasing sequence. The next difference is 16; and the next element, 33.

Differences can be negative as well as positive as in the sequence:

$$34 \quad 27 \quad 21 \quad 16 \quad 12 \quad \underline{\hspace{1cm}}$$

The successive differences: -7, -6, -5, -4, indicate that the next difference would be -3. Thus, the next element would be 12 - 3 or 9.

Some sequences do not depend on numeric relationships. For example,

> AB   DC   EF   HG   IJ   _____

is simply the alphabet with every other pair of letters reversed. Thus, since the pair IJ is in correct order, the next element in the sequence will be the next pair, KL, reversed or LK.

As the difficulty increases, you will be challenged to find more complex relationships. For example, given the following sequence:

> 2   3   5   8   13   _____

the differences between these elements are 1,2,3,5. These do not follow an obvious relationship. Here, beginning with 2 and 3, each following number is the sum of the two previous elements. Thus 2 + 3 = 5, 3 + 5 = 8, etc. Therefore, the next element in the sequence is 8 + 13 = 21.

Word Chains

A Word Chain exercise challenges verbal fluency, word recognition, and working memory. Verbal fluency is especially important in "finding the word" in everyday life. You are asked to find a sequence of words leading from a starting word to a target word. Each word in the sequence is obtained by changing one letter of the previous word. The number of blank lines between the start and the target indicate the number of words to be found in the sequence from the start to the target.

In the following example, given "stick" as the start and "click" as the target, the "t" in "stick" can be changed to "l" to obtain "slick" and then the "s" in "slick" can be changed to "c" to obtain the target "click." In the exercises, this would appear as

stick	that has the solution	stick
_____		_slick_
click		click

46

In some cases, words will pop into mind with little effort. If this doesn't happen, try changing one of the letters in the previous word in the sequence to match a letter in the target. There may be more than one solution to the exercise. For example, the following two chains lead from "head" to "feet."

head	head
heat	_heed_
feat	_feed_
feet	feet

If the number of intermediate words between the start and the target is less than the number of letters which are different between the start and target, then a solution can be found by simply changing one letter at a time to match a letter in the target. (See the above example.) Otherwise, you will have to do some guessing! In this case it may help to try working up from the target as well as down from the start. The following gives a chain from "fish" to "worm" requiring four intermediate words. (Note that the "e" in "wise" is not a letter in the target.)

fish

wish

wise

wire

wore

worm.

Rotations

A Rotations exercise challenges your visual working memory, visual acuity and the ability to mentally manipulate images. This ability is important whenever you have to make sense of visual information that may be presented in a new manner such as when driving or going down the aisles of a supermarket. Each exercise asks you to determine which images can be derived from a given image by simply rotating the image around its center without "reflecting" it (as it would appear if you held it up to a mirror). Another way of understanding a reflection is to imagine flipping the image over like a pancake.

In each exercise you select which images at the right of a line are rotations of the image at the left of the line. When the image of dove A in Example 1 is rotated slightly in a clockwise direction as indicated by the arrow, it is the same as the image at the left. Image B is the same image "standing on its head." All of the lettered images are rotations of the image at the left.

It may help to select one feature of the initial image, such as the head of the dove, which occurs on one side of the image but not the other. Then mentally rotate the image to be matched so that it is upright in the same way that the initial image is upright. Then determine if the selected feature is on the same side. All of the images A through D have their heads on the same side as the image at the left if they are rotated into an upright position.

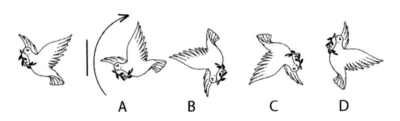

Example 1

If you apply this strategy to the images in Example 2, it is obvious that the head in image 1 is on the opposite side compared to the head of the initial image. This is because image 1 is a reflection of the initial image. Applying this strategy to images 2 through 5, you will see that only image 4 will have the head on the left when rotated into an upright position. Images 2, 3 and 5 are reflections of the initial image.

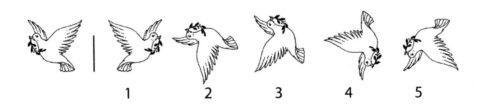

Example 2

Calculations

A Calculations exercise challenges your arithmetic abilities as well as concentration and attention. Try to work as quickly as possible. Also, try to avoid writing carries and borrows on the paper. This will give your short term memory and working memory extra exercise. A typical exercise will appear as:

50860	83782	67426	39734	36250
24719	37120	67207	97627	21201

63045	77049	27744	72031	95031
-51970	-30083	-10240	-38284	-23867

Finding Words

This is for the Scrabble fans! Finding words that can be spelled from the letters of a given word is good exercise for word fluency and processing speed. Limit your time to three minutes. A typical exercise will appear as:

Find as many words of three letters or more that can be made from the letters of the following word. (Time limit - 3 minutes)

AGILITY

_____   _____

_____   _____

_____   _____

_____   _____

_____   _____

Some of the answers are: **LAITY, TAIL, GAIT, GILT, TAG, LAG, and GAY.**

Symbol Counting

Counting symbols arranged in a random field gives important exercise for visual discrimination in the presence of distracters. This is something everyone driving a car into an intersection must be able to do very quickly! While you can likely increase your accuracy by running your finger across the page, avoid this if you can. Visually scanning a larger field of view will bring greater benefit. An example of this exercise is:

Count the number of each symbol.

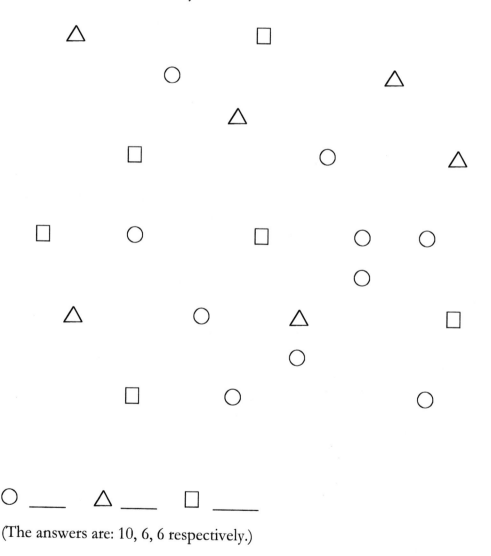

(The answers are: 10, 6, 6 respectively.)

Naming

Naming exercises require finding names of a particular class, such as flowers. This can help finding that word on the tip of your tongue. It may be useful to think of categories of items and then fill in the details. For example, when asked to name animals, you might think of pets, farm animals, wild animals, etc. and then fill in "cat", "dog", "cow", "horse", "lion", "elephant", etc. Doing this makes use of associations in your semantic memory.

Word Matrix

The Word Matrix exercise challenges visual perception and working memory and requires your brain to filter out distractions. You are asked to find the numbered words within the letters of the matrix. The words within the matrix can be spelled backwards or forwards, up or down, and diagonally. In the example, the solution is given with the words enclosed in rounded boxes.

Sometimes you will see a given word as a whole; it may seem to spring out of the matrix at you! At other times when you may have more difficulty, it may help to search for the first letter of the target word and, when the first letter is found, to look at the 8 letters surrounding that letter. If one of the 8 letters is the second letter of the target word, continue in the direction of the second letter looking for the third letter, etc. When this doesn't work, you might try searching for a short string of the target word.

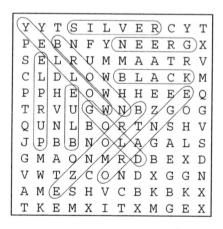

1. BLACK	6. BLUE
2. BRONZE	7. BROWN
3. GREEN	8. ORANGE
4. PURPLE	9. SILVER
5. YELLOW	10. GOLD

Coding

A Coding exercise challenges your visual perception and short term memory. You are required to decode a quote encoded in visual figures or icons by locating these figures in a table. The more icon-letter associations you can remember, the faster your processing speed will be.

In some cases you will be able to identify a word in the quote by context without having to decode it. However, for the greatest benefit, do at least check out your guesses by decoding the words. An example is:

Coding: Decode the message using the code table.

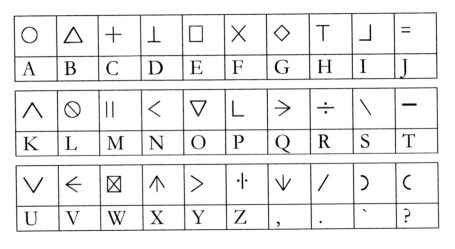

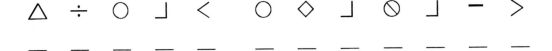

By using the code table, you can see that the symbol △ corresponds to the letter B; the symbol ÷ to the letter R, etc. The decoded message is BRAIN AGILITY.

Shopping List and To-Do List

One of these memory exercises will be given each day. Take time to read the list aloud, cover it with your hand, and repeat as much as you can aloud. Do this three times. It may help if you identify categories among the items such as meat, vegetables, etc. Other helpful strategies are to visualize the items as they might be arranged in a familiar supermarket or to visualize yourself doing the activities of the to-do list as you might do them during the day. You will be asked to write the list immediately after committing it to memory and then again at the end of the exercises for the day.

Fact of the Day

One of these memory exercises will be given each day. As with the Shopping and To-Do Lists, take time to read the fact aloud, cover it with your hand and repeat as much as you can. Do this three times. It may be helpful to visualize the information of the fact and to relate it to something in your current life. You will be asked to write the fact immediately after committing it to memory and then again at the end of the exercises for the day.

Schedules

This exercise involves working with airline schedules to calculate time differences between cities and the length of flights -- a real world problem that challenges your arithmetic abilities, working memory, concentration, and logical abilities. Because this is the most complex of the exercises, a more detailed explanation of strategies for solving it is given than for the other exercises.

The schedule for each exercise is divided into two parts: an airline schedule on the left and a table of cities, airport codes and time zones on the right. The airline schedule gives origin, destination, departure time, arrival time, and flight number. Notice that the origin and destination codes in the schedule are codes for the cities in the table on the right.

orig	dest	depart	arrive	flt#
DTW	SFO	9:22a	11:25a	343
DTW	SFO	12:15p	2:22p	345
DTW	SFO	7:39p	9:51p	347
FRA	DTW	10:20a	1:55p	51
SFO	NRT	12:00p	4:30p*	27

city	code	time
Detroit	DTW	GMT-5
Frankfurt	FRA	GMT+1
San Francisco	SFO	GMT-8
Tokyo	NRT	GMT+9

* next day

Working with Time Zones

You may likely work with time zones when telephoning someone in another area of the country or world. Also, planning to watch a live television program being broadcast from another part of the country requires working with differences between time zones. The continental United States is divided into four time zones: Eastern, Central, Mountain, and Pacific. Beginning with Eastern Time, each time zone is "one hour ahead" of the next time zone traveling west.

Internationally there are 24 time zones which divide the time for the whole planet. Each of these zones is given an offset relative to Greenwich, England. The time in Greenwich is called "Greenwich Mean Time" (GMT) or "Universal Time." The offset, relative to Greenwich, for each time zone is the number of hours that zone is ahead of or behind Greenwich, England. The following diagram gives the offset for a number of major world cities. All of the cities you will have to deal with in the exercises are listed in this diagram. The offsets for the cities are given in the "time" column of each schedule exercise. Although daylight savings time will produce some changes in this diagram, daylight savings time will not be considered in any of the exercises.

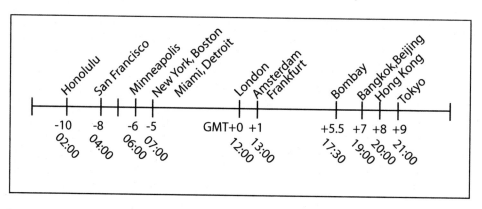

London is at GMT+0, which means that it has the same time as Greenwich. The time zones to the right of London are ahead of London by the given number of hours. Thus Amsterdam is 1 hour ahead of London. When it is noon in London, it is 1:00pm in Amsterdam. The time zones to the left of London are behind London by the given number of hours. New York, which is in Eastern Standard Time, is 5 hours behind London. When it is 12:00pm in London, it is 7:00am in New York. If it is 9:00am in London and you want to telephone someone in New York, you need to know that it is 4:00am in New York.

Keeping track of time zones is often made easier by using the 24 hour time notation. Thus 1:00pm is written as 13:00 (12:00 + 1 hour). Looking at the diagram, you can see that Hong Kong is at GMT+8 or 8 hours ahead of London. Thus when it is 12:00 (12:00pm) in London, it is 12:00 + 8 or 20:00 (8:00pm) in Hong Kong.

To calculate time differences between a city that is ahead of London and one which is behind London requires adding the offsets. For example to calculate the time in Tokyo when it is 1:00pm or 13:00 in San Francisco, first note in the table that London is 8 hours ahead of San Francisco, and Tokyo is 9 hours ahead of London. This means that Tokyo is 9 + 8 =17 hours ahead of San Francisco. This can be seen by looking at the diagram.

Thus, when flight 27 in the table departs, it is 12:00pm in San Francisco. At this moment it is 12:00 + 17 = 29:00 in Tokyo. Of course 29:00 is not a valid time. That 29:00 is greater than 24:00 means that we have gone beyond midnight (24:00). Therefore we have to subtract 24:00 from 29:00 to get 05:00. Because we have gone past midnight, it is 5:00am the next day. Thus, when it is 12:00 in San Francisco, it is five o'clock in the morning in Tokyo -- the next day. Some people find it easier to calculate 12:00pm + 12 to reach midnight and then to add the remaining 5 hours to midnight to obtain 5:00am the next day. Do whatever works best for you.

The schedule exercises included in Day 1 to Day 8 of the exercises require only calculating the time differences between cities. You may wish to wait until you have completed these before reading the following discussion of how to calculate the length of a flight.

Calculating the Length of a Flight

orig	dest	depart	arrive	flt#
DTW	SFO	9:22a	11:25a	343
DTW	SFO	12:15p	2:22p	345
DTW	SFO	7:39p	9:51p	347
FRA	DTW	10:20a	1:55p	51
SFO	NRT	12:00p	4:30p*	27

city	code	time
Detroit	DTW	GMT-5
Frankfurt	FRA	GMT+1
San Francisco	SFO	GMT-8
Tokyo	NRT	GMT+9

* next day

In order to calculate the length of a flight, we must subtract the time an airplane takes off from the time it lands. For example, if we are on flight 343 from Detroit to San Francisco, we leave at 9:22am and arrive at 11:25am. At first glance this might seem as if the length of the flight is 2 hours and 3 minutes. However, the departure and arrival times are in the local times of the origin and destination cities respectively. To calculate the length of a flight we must first convert the departure time to the time zone of the destination city and then subtract this from the arrival time. Considering the time differences, we know that the time in San Francisco when flight 343 departs is 9:22am - 3 hours or 6:22am. Thus the length of the flight is actually 11:25am - 6:22am or 5 hours and 3 minutes.

If we are traveling from Frankfort to Detroit on flight 51, we leave at 10:20am and arrive at 1:55pm. Considering the differences between the time zones, we know that when we take off in Frankfort it is 4:20am in Detroit. Thus the length of the flight is the time from 4:20am until 1:55pm or 9 hours and 35 minutes. To calculate time in the air for a multi-leg trip, calculate the time for each leg using these procedures and then add the times.

Calculating Total Travel Time

When calculating total travel time, you only need the departure time from the initial origin and the arrival time at the final destination. However, when there are multiple legs, you will need to use the schedule to identify the appropriate connecting flights in order to determine the final arrival time.

orig	dest	depart	arrive	flt#
DTW	SFO	9:22a	11:25a	343
DTW	SFO	12:15p	2:22p	345
DTW	SFO	7:39p	9:51p	347
FRA	DTW	10:20a	1:55p	51
SFO	NRT	12:00p	4:30p*	27

city	code	time
Detroit	DTW	GMT-5
Frankfurt	FRA	GMT+1
San Francisco	SFO	GMT-8
Tokyo	NRT	GMT+9

* next day

To calculate the total travel time from Frankfurt to San Francisco, first note that the only flight out of Frankfort is flight 51. Since this flight arrives at 1:55 pm, the next flight from Detroit to San Francisco is flight 347. You now know the departure time from Frankfurt and the arrival time in San Francisco. Since Frankfurt is GMT+1 and San Francisco GMT-8, when the flight leaves Frankfurt, the local time in San Francisco is 10:20am - 9 hours or 01:20am. Since the arrival time in San Francisco is 9:51pm or 21:51, the total travel time is 21:51 - 01:20 = 20:31 or 20 hours and 31 minutes. Since you are only concerned with total travel time, you do not need to consider flight time from Frankfort to Detroit, layover time in Detroit, or flight time from Detroit to San Francisco.

Additional Points

In some cases the schedule will indicate that a time is "next day." For example, flight 27 from San Francisco to Tokyo leaves at 12:00pm and arrives in Tokyo at 04:30pm or 16:30 the next day. To calculate the time in the air, first note that San Francisco is GMT-8 and Tokyo GMT+9. When it is 12:00pm in San Francisco, it is 17 hours later in Tokyo. Thus when the flight leaves San Francisco, it is 12:00pm +17 hours = 29:00 or 29:00 - 24:00 = 05:00am in Tokyo. Thus the time in the air is arrival time minus departure time (adjusted to local time of destination) or 16:30 - 05:00 = 11:30 or 11 hours and 30 minutes.

Note that when adding and subtracting hours and minutes, if the sum of minutes is greater than 60, then for each 60 minutes 1 hour must be "carried" into the hour column. And if a "borrow" must be made from the hours column, this means borrowing 60 minutes. For example, calculating 11:25am plus 4 hours and 45 minutes = 11:25am + 4:45 = 16:10, (45 min. + 25 min. = 70 min. = 1 hour and 10 minutes.)

As noted above you can do the calculations without using the 24 hour notation. However, be sure to keep track of whether the calculated time is am or pm.

When doing the schedule exercises, do your best and refer back to this section when necessary. If an exercise takes more than 10 minutes, move on to the next. You will have exercised your brain in spite of not finding the answer. If you want, go back to it later.

The Brain Agility Exercises 10

Brain Agility Exercises

I. Complete the following sequences.

1	3	5	7	9	_11_
23	19	15	11	7	_3_
4	8	12	16	20	_24_
3	4	6	9	13	_18_
20	19	17	14	10	_15_ ✓ _5_

Time: min. _5_ sec._____

II. Shopping List

Remember as much as you can of this shopping list by reading it aloud, covering it with your hand and saying aloud as many of the items as you can. Repeat this three times. It may help to identify categories in the items such as meat or vegetables.

trout
celery
milk
green peppers
tomatoes
grapefruit
lettuce
cereal
sausage
pasta sauce

III. Fact of the Day (Read aloud, cover, and say aloud -- three times.)

Life expectancy in the United States in 1901 was 49 years.
At the end of the century it was 77 years, an increase of 57%.

Day 1   Brain Agility Exercises

IV. Write as many of the Shopping List items as you can remember.

celery   _tomatoes_

green peppers   _trout_

lettuce   _cereal_

eggs   _pasta sauce_

milk

V. Write as much as you can of the Fact of the Day.

Life expectancy in the US in 1901 was 49 years. At the end of the century it was 77 years, an increase of 57%

VI. Word Chains
Complete the following word chains. Beginning with the first word, change one letter at a time to create a new word ending with the bottom word.

snare	mall	pile	boar
_____	_____	_____	_____
_____	_____	_____	_____
sport	bane	none	meat

Time: min. ____ sec. ____

VII. Find the figures which are rotations and not reflections of the figure
     at the left of each line. *ugh !!!*

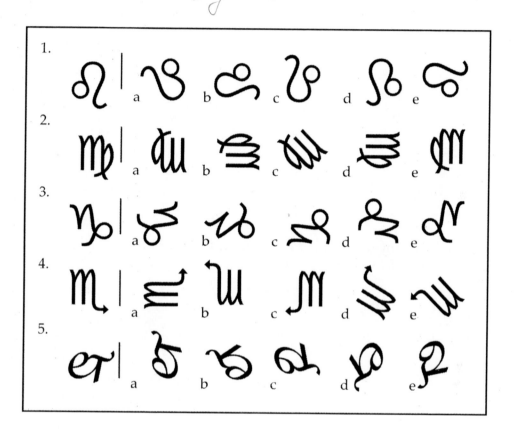

1)_____ 2)_____ 3)_____ 4)_____ 5)_____

Time: min. ____ sec. ____

VIII. Calculate the following:

| 71785 | 12853 | 1977 | 51220 | 33390 |
| 17708 | 38251 | 8309 | 68235 | 55493 |

| 47004 | 53158 | 48233 | 96881 | 27759 |
| 45762 | 88654 | 21624 | 14031 | 60243 |

Time: min. _____ sec. _____

IX. Find as many words of three letters or more which can be made from the letters of the following word. (Time limit - 3 minutes)

BRAIN

bra _____   _____
rain _____   _____
bran _____   _____
ran _____   _____
air _____   _____
? rabi _____   _____
_____   _____

Brain Agility Exercises

X. Count the number of each symbol.

```
        +               O               O
            +       +
            -                       +
    O               + -
    -           O       O       +
    -       -       -           -
        + -             O  +    O
        O
            O           O  -     +
                O           O

    O                   -           -


+ _9_   - _11_   O _13_
```

Time: min. _____sec. _40_

65

XI. Name as many foods as you can in one minute.

bananas	yogurt
walnuts	butter
bread	lettuce
pita	celery
tomato	cranberries
orange	peanut butter
apple	
meat	
eggs	
milk	

XII. Write as many of the Shopping List items as you can remember.

celery	milk
grapefruit	cereal
tomatoes	sauce
green peppers	trout
eggs	

XIII. Write as much as you can of the Fact of the Day.

Life expectancy in 1901 was 49 yr
at the end of the century it was 77.
increase of 57%.

Brain Agility Exercises

I. Word Matrix (Find the following words in the matrix.)

1. BEAR
2. ELEPHANT
3. GORILLA
4. LEOPARD
5. LION
6. PANTHER
7. ZEBRA
8. MONKEY

```
R U O J E G R O W G
J B J A R O G T S T
X Z U I A R Z T T P
L N Y R E I E N E R
Y E O E B L B A N E
V E O I C L R H I H
Z N K P L A A P X T
T G K N A Z W E M N
W T U R O R G L F A
I J E D G M D E N P
```

Time: min. _____ sec. _____

II. To-Do List (Read aloud, cover, repeat aloud -- three times.)

register for evening class
concert tonight
dental appointment
return library books
buy new printer cartridge
go to talk on health insurance
sign up for volunteer project

III. Fact of the Day (Read aloud, cover, and say aloud -- three times.)

Mensa is an international society for those who score within the top 2% on a standardized intelligence test.

IV. Write as many of the To-Do list items as you can remember.

Reg for evening class

Dental app.

Concert tonight

cartrige

Health insurance

Volunteer

V. Write as much as you can of the Fact of the Day.

Mensa is an internat'l society for those who score over 2% on intelligence test

VI. Schedule

orig	dest	depart	arrive	flt#
SEA	MSP	12:50a	5:53a	154
SEA	MSP	7:00a	12:16p	806
SEA	MSP	8:55a	2:07p	158
SEA	MSP	12:20p	5:33p	170
SEA	MSP	3:11p	9:23p	164
MSP	JFK	7:00a	10:33a	362
MSP	JFK	12:55p	4:34p	734
MSP	JFK	7:00p	10:35p	198

city	code	time
Seattle	SEA	GMT-8
Minneapolis	MSP	GMT-6
New York	JFK	GMT-5

a) When it is 7:00am in Seattle, what time is it in New York?___ 10:00 AM

b) When it is 12:55pm in Minneapolis, what time is it in Seattle?_____

Time: min. _____ sec. _____

Brain Agility Exercises

VII. Find the figures which are <u>rotations</u> and not reflections of the figure at the left of each line.

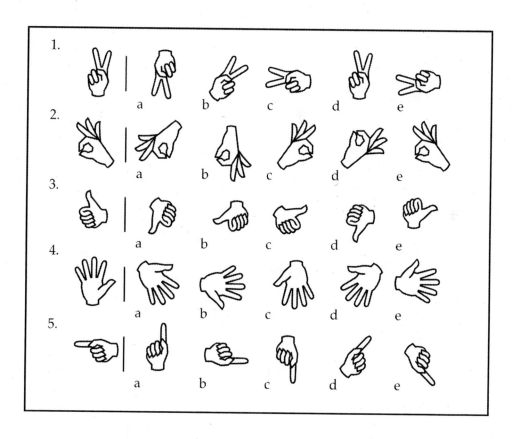

1)_____ 2)_____ 3)_____ 4)_____ 5)_____

Time: min. ____ sec. ____

VIII. Calculate the following:

72238	47563	73825	97967	88557
95166	63536	99216	73238	16399

69579	10740	36057	87363	47197
16037	40400	74140	60504	15700

Time: min. _____ sec. _____

IX. Find as many words of three letters or more which can be made from the letters of the following word. (Time limit - 3 minutes)

SWEDEN

_____   _____

_____   _____

_____   _____

_____   _____

_____   _____

_____   _____

_____   _____

X. Coding: Decode the message using the code table.

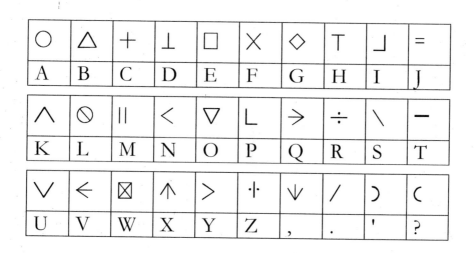

⊤ □   ⊠ ⊤ ▽   ⊤ □ \ ⌐ ─ ○ ─ □ \   ⌐ \
H E   W H O   H E S I T A T E S   I S

\ ▽ ‖ □ ─ ⌐ ‖ □ \   \ ○ ← □ ⊥ /
S O M E T I M E S   S A V E D .

-- James Thurber

Time: min. 4 sec. ____

XI. Name as many animals as you can in one minute.

_____   _____

_____   _____

_____   _____

_____   _____

_____   _____

_____   _____

_____   _____

_____   _____

XII. Write as many of the To-Do list items as you can remember.

_____

_____

_____

_____

_____

_____

_____

XIII. Write as much as you can of the Fact of the Day.

_____

_____

_____

_____

I. Word Matrix (Find the following words in the matrix.)

1. CHEESE
2. CHICKEN
3. LENTILS
4. MILK
5. OATMEAL
6. PORK
7. PRUNES
8. RICE

```
C H E E S E J Y S
H C P I B S O N L
A X K H E A E R I
Z N F N T K I M T
B B U M C C W D N
Y R E I E T O M E
P A H M G F J I L
L C P O R K E L P
I W Q H U I Q K R
```

Time: min. ____ sec. ____

II. Shopping List (Read aloud, cover, repeat aloud -- three times.)

butter
applesauce
toothpaste
apricots
oatmeal
red snapper
paper toweling
broccoli
coffee
cereal

III. Fact of the Day (Read aloud, cover, and say aloud -- three times.)

As of January 2007, approximately 1,094,000,000 people worldwide use the Internet according to Internet World Stats.

IV. Write as many of the Shopping List items as you can remember.

_____   _____

_____   _____

_____   _____

_____   _____

_____   _____

V. Write as much as you can of the Fact of the Day.

_____

_____

_____

_____

VI. Word Chains

Complete the following word chains.

look	fill	stick	stars
____	____	____	____
____	____	____	____
fool	wine	spice	spark

Time: min. ____ sec. ____

Brain Agility Exercises

VII. Coding: Decode the message using the code table.

○	△	+	⊥	□	X	◇	T	⌐	=
A	B	C	D	E	F	G	H	I	J

∧	⊘	‖	<	∇	L	→	÷	\	—
K	L	M	N	O	P	Q	R	S	T

∨	←	⊠	↑	>	·|·	↓	/	)	(
U	V	W	X	Y	Z	,	.	'	?

○ ◇ □   ⌐ \   ○   T ⌐ ◇ T

— — —   — —   —   — — — —

L ÷ ⌐ + □   — ∇   L ○ >

— — — — —   — —   — — —

X ∇ ÷   ‖ ○ — ∨ ÷ ⌐ — > /

— — —   — — — — — — — — —

-- Tom Stoppard

Time: min. _____sec._____

VIII. Schedule

orig	dest	depart	arrive	flt#
BOS	DTW	7:06a	9:23a	377
BOS	DTW	9:04a	11:25a	375
BOS	DTW	11:59a	2:14p	1195
BOS	DTW	2:37p	4:54p	381
BOS	DTW	4:12p	6:29p	207
BOS	DTW	5:48p	8:08p	373
BOS	DTW	7:37p	9:49p	379
DTW	SFO	9:22a	11:25a	343
DTW	SFO	12:15p	2:22p	345
DTW	SFO	7:39p	9:51p	347

city	code	time
Boston	BOS	GMT-5
Detroit	DTW	GMT-5
San Francisco	SFO	GMT-8

a) When it is 9:04am in Boston, what time is it in San Francisco?_____

b) What is the time in Detroit when it is 2:22pm in San Francisco?_____

Time: min. _____sec._____

IX. Complete the following sequences.

10	14	18	22	26	_____
3	5	8	12	17	_____
47	43	39	35	31	_____
9	14	12	17	15	_____
19	13	17	11	15	_____

Time: min. _____sec._____

X. Count the number of each symbol.

◯ ___ △ ___ □ ___   Time: min. _____sec._____

XI. Name as many trees as you can in one minute.

_____   _____

_____   _____

_____   _____

_____   _____

_____   _____

_____   _____

_____   _____

_____   _____

_____   _____

XII. Write as many of the Shopping List items as you can remember.

_____   _____

_____   _____

_____   _____

_____   _____

_____   _____

XIII. Write as much as you can of the Fact of the Day.

_____

_____

_____

_____

I. Complete the following sequences.

6	11	17	24	32	_____
26	24	21	17	12	_____
9	11	15	21	29	_____
29	27	24	20	15	_____
7	11	12	16	17	_____

Time: min. _____sec._____

II. Shopping List(Read aloud, cover, repeat aloud -- three times.)

tea
cream
grapes
acorn squash
ham
potato chips
bok choy
cheese
cantaloupe
tomato soup

III. Fact of the Day (Read aloud, cover, and say aloud -- three times.)

Guglielmo Marconi (1874-1937) was the inventor of wireless telegraphy, forerunner of the radio, for which he shared the 1909 Nobel Prize in Physics.

IV. Write as many of the Shopping List items as you can remember.

_____   _____

_____   _____

_____   _____

_____   _____

_____   _____

V. Write as much as you can of the Fact of the Day.

_____

_____

_____

_____

VI. Word Chains

goat   peak   boil   half

_____   _____   _____   _____

_____   _____   _____   _____

colt   head   cook   bake

Time: min. _____ sec. _____

VII. Find the figures which are rotations and not reflections of the figure at the left of each line.

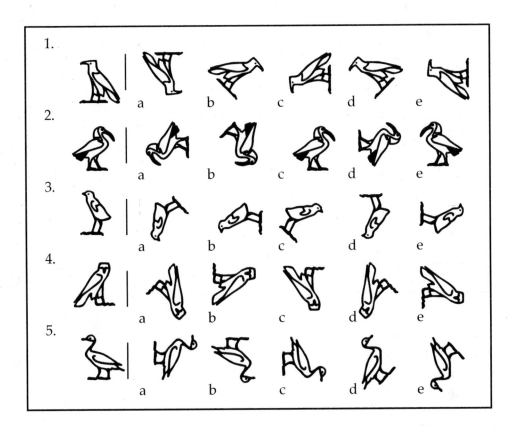

1)_____ 2)_____ 3)_____ 4)_____ 5)_____

Time: min. _____sec._____

VIII. Calculate the following:

63554	59386	43587	42777	61443
36176	21306	83368	87180	47293

38637	96898	60069	57823	56086
16872	14241	84297	87208	86513

Time: min. _____ sec. _____

IX. Find as many words of three letters or more which can be made from the letters of the following word. (Time limit - 3 minutes)

EXERCISE

_____   _____

_____   _____

_____   _____

_____   _____

_____   _____

_____   _____

_____   _____

Brain Agility Exercises

X. Count the number of each symbol.

%   % $

$ &

%   &   %   &

$ $ $

& $

&   %   %

& $ $ $

$

%   % $ %

% $ $ $

$ $ &

% $ % $

$___ %___&___

Time: min. _____sec._____

XI. Name as many flowers as you can in one minute.

_____	_____
_____	_____
_____	_____
_____	_____
_____	_____
_____	_____
_____	_____

XII. Write as many of the Shopping List items as you can remember.

_____	_____
_____	_____
_____	_____
_____	_____
_____	_____

XIII. Write as much as you can of the Fact of the Day.

_____

_____

_____

_____

Brain Agility Exercises

I. Word Matrix (Find the following words in the matrix.)

1. CABINET
2. CARPET
3. CHAIR
4. COUCH
5. DESK
6. DRESSER
7. LAMP
8. STOOL
9. TABLE
10. ROCKER

```
L L T C R Q I W Y Y
K A A O L E K O R K
N M B U D O K S F I
S P L C X R O C E O
K U E H V W I T O D
O A F U H H A A S R
P C A B I N E T H V
B C A R P E T U P C
O L D R E S S E R T
G J F A J Q Q J V A
```

Time: min. ____ sec. ____

II. To-Do List(Read aloud, cover, repeat aloud -- three times.)

take clothes to cleaner
cancel airline tickets
write letter to congressional reps
put out trash
make appointment with doctor
take dog to veterinarian
go to post office

III. Fact of the Day (Read aloud, cover, and say aloud -- three times.)

In the United States, Mothers' Day was originally conceived by social activist Julia Ward Howe during the American Civil War with a call to unite women against war.

IV. Write as many of the To-Do list items as you can remember.

_____

_____

_____

_____

_____

_____

_____

V. Write as much as you can of the Fact of the Day.

_____

_____

_____

_____

VI. Schedule

orig	dest	depart	arrive	flt#
MIA	MSP	7:30a	10:26a	571
MIA	MSP	12:57p	3:50p	573
MIA	MSP	5:22p	8:21p	575
MSP	SEA	5:23p	7:07p	161
MSP	SEA	9:40p	11:24p	165

city	code	time
Miami	MIA	GMT-5
Minneapolis	MSP	GMT-6
Seattle	SEA	GMT-8

a) If it is 11:24pm in Seattle, what time is it in Miami?_____

b) What is the time in Seattle when flight 161 leaves Minneapolis?_____

c) What is the time in Minneapolis when flight 573 leaves Miami?_____

Time: min. _____sec._____

Brain Agility Exercises

VII. Find the figures which are rotations and not reflections of the figure at the left of each line.

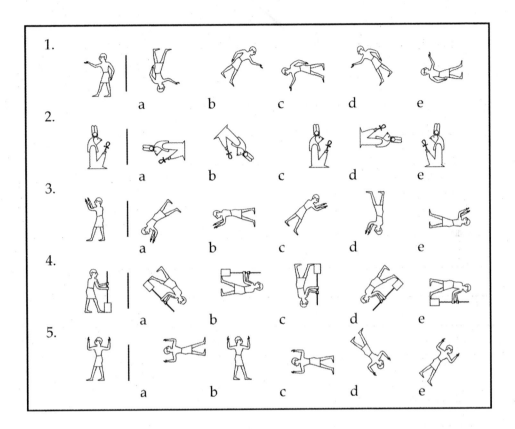

1.

    a   b   c   d   e

2.

    a   b   c   d   e

3.

    a   b   c   d   e

4.

    a   b   c   d   e

5.

    a   b   c   d   e

1)_____ 2)_____ 3)_____ 4)_____ 5)_____

Time: min. ____ sec. ____

VIII. Calculate the following:

31799	23596	87549	69912	64138
77191	75640	60239	49170	12975

98750	42768	47141	72839	95855
77599	21393	23794	59172	96162

Time: min. _____ sec. _____

IX. Find as many words of three letters or more which can be made from the letters of the following word. (Time limit - 3 minutes)

EUROPE

_____	_____
_____	_____
_____	_____
_____	_____
_____	_____
_____	_____
_____	_____

Brain Agility Exercises

X. Coding: Decode the message using the code table.

○	△	+	⊥	□	✕	◇	T	⌐	=
A	B	C	D	E	F	G	H	I	J

∧	⊘	‖	<	▽	L	→	÷	\	−
K	L	M	N	O	P	Q	R	S	T

∨	⇐	⊠	↑	>	·∤·	↓	/	)	(
U	V	W	X	Y	Z	,	.	'	?

○ ⊘ ⊘   ⊠ ▽ ∨ ⊘ ⊥   ⊘ ⌐ ⇐ □

A L L   W O U L D   L I V E

⊘ ▽ < ◇ ↓   △ ∨ −   < ▽ < □

L O N G ,   B U T   N O N E

⊠ ▽ ∨ ⊘ ⊥   △ □   ▽ ⊘ ⊥ /

W O U L D   B E   O L D .

-- Benjamin Franklin

Time: min. ____ sec. ____

XI. Name as many countries as you can in one minute.

_____   _____

_____   _____

_____   _____

_____   _____

_____   _____

_____   _____

_____   _____

_____   _____

XII. Write as many of the To-Do list items as you can remember.

_____

_____

_____

_____

_____

_____

_____

XIII. Write as much as you can of the Fact of the Day.

_____

_____

_____

_____

Brain Agility Exercises

I. Word Matrix (Find the following words in the matrix.)

1. APPLE
2. ASPEN
3. BEECH
4. GINKO
5. REDWOOD
6. SYCAMORE
7. WALNUT
8. CHESTNUT

```
I  B  H  B  T  J  X  V  N  U
H  F  E  N  N  U  D  M  S  K
I  R  N  R  M  O  N  D  T  Q
O  A  R  E  O  G  V  L  E  W
K  D  P  W  P  M  I  H  A  K
D  Y  D  P  Q  S  A  N  F  W
J  E  C  F  L  L  A  C  K  N
R  T  H  C  E  E  B  T  Y  O
K  T  U  N  T  S  E  H  C  S
H  W  O  N  E  S  H  I  I  E
```

Time: min. _____ sec. _____

II. Shopping List(Read aloud, cover, repeat aloud -- three times.)

onions
broccoli
salmon
peanut butter
ground beef
orange juice
spaghetti sauce
cereal
green peppers
eggplant

III. Fact of the Day (Read aloud, cover, and say aloud -- three times.)

The human brain contains more than 100 billion neurons, each linked to as many as 10,000 others.

IV. Write as many of the Shopping List items as you can remember.

_____   _____

_____   _____

_____   _____

_____   _____

_____   _____

V. Write as much as you can of the Fact of the Day.

_____

_____

_____

_____

VI. Word Chains

slick   clock   date

_____   _____   _____

_____   _____   _____

space   snack   _____

                                      pits

Time: min. _____ sec. _____

VII. Coding: Decode the message using the code table.

○	△	+	⊥	□	✕	◇	⊤	⌐	=
A	B	C	D	E	F	G	H	I	J

∧	⊘	∥	<	▽	L	→	÷	\	—
K	L	M	N	O	P	Q	R	S	T

∨	←	⊠	↑	>	·⊦	↓	/	)	(
U	V	W	X	Y	Z	,	.	'	?

∥   >   ▽   <   □   ÷   □   ◇   ÷   □   —
__ __ __ __ __ __ __ __ __ __ __

⌐   <   ⊘   ⌐   ✕   □   ⌐   \
__ __ __ __ __ __ __ __

—   ⊤   ○   —   ⌐   ○   ∥   <   ▽   —
__ __ __ __ __ __ __ __ __ __

\   ▽   ∥   □   ▽   <   □   □   ⊘   \   □   /
__ __ __ __ __ __ __ __ __ __ __

-- Woody Allen

Time: min. _____ sec. _____

93

VIII. Schedule

orig	dest	depart	arrive	flt#
DTW	BOS	6:26a	8:14a	382
DTW	BOS	8:48a	10:36a	384
DTW	BOS	10:32a	12:19p	372
DTW	BOS	1:32p	3:22p	386
DTW	BOS	3:10p	5:02p	370
DTW	BOS	4:57p	6:43p	276
DTW	BOS	7:01p	8:48p	378
DTW	BOS	9:05p	10:55p	1728
DTW	BOS	9:06p	10:52p	278
SEA	DTW	8:40a	3:54p	210
SEA	DTW	12:30p	7:40p	250
SEA	DTW	10:06p	5:06a*	208

city	code	time
Boston	BOS	GMT-5
Detroit	DTW	GMT-5
Seattle	SEA	GMT-8

* next day

a) If you must be in Boston by 7:00pm, what is the latest time you can leave Detroit?_____

b) When flight 378 arrives in Boston, what is the time in Seattle?_____

c) When flight 250 leaves Seattle, what is the time in Detroit?_____

Time: min. _____sec._____

IX. Complete the following sequences.

8	9	11	14	18	_____
11	13	17	25	41	_____
10	12	8	10	6	_____
21	19	16	12	7	_____
87	81	75	69	63	_____

Time: min. _____sec._____

Brain Agility Exercises

Day 6

X. Count the number of each symbol.

△ _____ ☐ _____ ◇ _____

Time: min. _____ sec. _____

95

XI. Name as many states as you can in one minute.

_____   _____

_____   _____

_____   _____

_____   _____

_____   _____

_____   _____

_____   _____

_____   _____

_____   _____

_____   _____

XII. Write as many of the Shopping List items as you can remember.

_____   _____

_____   _____

_____   _____

_____   _____

_____   _____

XIII. Write as much as you can of the Fact of the Day.

_____

_____

_____

_____

I. Complete the following sequences.

9	12	10	13	11	_____
10	12	10	13	10	_____
2	4	8	16	32	_____
16	12	16	13	16	_____
3	7	12	18	25	_____

Time: min. _____sec._____

II. Shopping List(Read aloud, cover, repeat aloud -- three times.)

coffee
clam chowder
apples
corn
sugar
grapefruit
ice cream
grapes
chicken
acorn squash

III. Fact of the Day (Read aloud, cover, and say aloud -- three times.)

The sun is 93 million miles from the earth. It takes light over 8 minutes to travel from the sun to the earth.

IV. Write as many of the Shopping List items as you can remember.

_____	_____
_____	_____
_____	_____
_____	_____
_____	_____

V. Write as much as you can of the Fact of the Day.

_____

_____

_____

_____

VI. Word Chains

talk	bill	rise
____	____	____
____	____	____
yell	half	____
		fall

Time: min. _____ sec. _____

Brain Agility Exercises

Day 7

VII. Find the figures which are rotations and not reflections of the figure at the left of each line.

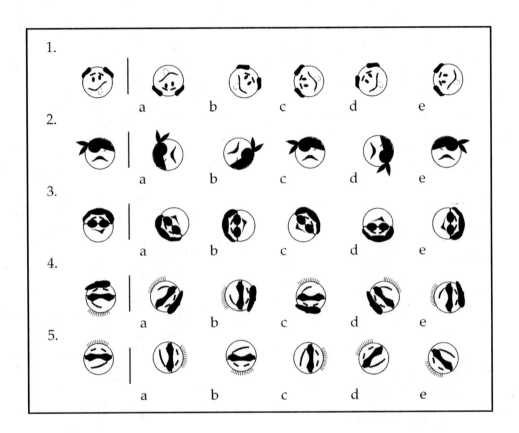

1) _____ 2) _____ 3) _____ 4) _____ 5) _____

Time: min. _____ sec. _____

VIII. Calculate the following:

66004	79198	67495	82348	81597
12590	87353	96358	29020	4194

31171	91220	24435	34119	48154
82396	46355	75834	16861	76509

Time: min. _____ sec. _____

IX. Find as many words of three letters or more which can be made from the letters of the following word. (Time limit - 3 minutes)

DIFFICULT

_____	_____
_____	_____
_____	_____
_____	_____
_____	_____
_____	_____
_____	_____

Brain Agility Exercises

X. Count the number of each symbol.

▽   □   △

△ _____ □ _____ ▽ _____

Time: min. _____ sec. _____

XI. Name as many presidents as you can in one minute.

_____	_____
_____	_____
_____	_____
_____	_____
_____	_____
_____	_____
_____	_____
_____	_____
_____	_____
_____	_____

XII. Write as many of the Shopping List items as you can remember.

_____	_____
_____	_____
_____	_____
_____	_____
_____	_____

XIII. Write as much as you can of the Fact of the Day.

_____

_____

_____

_____

Brain Agility Exercises

I. Word Matrix (Find the following words in the matrix.)

1. BELGIUM
2. CHILE
3. ENGLAND
4. INDIA
5. INDONESIA
6. JAPAN
7. NEPAL
8. SWITZERLAND
9. TIBET
10. THAILAND

```
N Q T H A I L A N D D C
L B M U I G L E B N H D
G N U A Q E W Q A R B N
J A E N Q J L L H I W A
A X I P D V R I N S D L
P R C X A E M D H C U G
A Z S T Z L O S A C P N
N B U T E N S I O H O E
I N I J E B D Y A H G V
Y W F S U N I X W S S H
S B I O I N X T I N V G
B A H X M V A U F K V G
```

Time: min. ____ sec. ____

II. To-Do List(Read aloud, cover, repeat aloud -- three times.)

register for evening class
special on TV tonight
go to brain agility class
doctor's appointment
do brain agility exercises
call plumber
renew newspaper

III. Fact of the Day (Read aloud, cover, and say aloud -- three times.)

A study in the Netherlands involving 800 healthy men and women aged 50 to 70 found over a 3-year period that a daily supplement of 800 micrograms of folic acid significantly improved memory and information processing.

IV. Write as many of the To-Do list items as you can remember.

_____

_____

_____

_____

_____

_____

_____

V. Write as much as you can of the Fact of the Day.

_____

_____

_____

_____

VI. Schedule

orig	dest	depart	arrive	flt#
DTW	SFO	9:22a	11:25a	343
DTW	SFO	12:15p	2:22p	345
DTW	SFO	7:39p	9:51p	347
JFK	DTW	9:02a	11:13a	898
JFK	DTW	12:35p	2:53p	894
JFK	DTW	4:11p	6:25p	896

city	code	time
Detroit	DTW	GMT-5
New York	JFK	GMT-5
San Francisco	SFO	GMT-8

a) If you cannot leave New York before noon, what is the earliest you can arrive in San Francisco?_____

b) When you arrive in San Francisco what is the time in New York?_____

c) When flight 347 leaves Detroit, what is the time in San Francisco?_____

Time: min. ____ sec. ____

Brain Agility Exercises

VII. Find the figures which are rotations and not reflections of the figure on the left of each line.

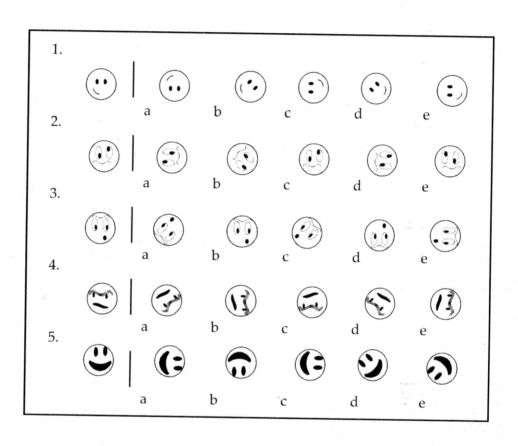

1)_____ 2)_____ 3)_____ 4)_____ 5)_____

Time: min. _____sec._____

VIII. Calculate the following:

| 24506 | 39164 | 25045 | 55487 | 12286 |
| 82481 | 62659 | 61551 | 65838 | 95028 |

| 58197 | 61471 | 36630 | 37346 | 76991 |
| 56173 | 37001 | 75967 | 37622 | 39243 |

Time: min. _____sec._____

IX. Find as many words of three letters or more which can be made from the letters of the following word. (Time limit - 3 minutes)

TRAVEL

_____   _____

_____   _____

_____   _____

_____   _____

_____   _____

_____   _____

_____   _____

X. Coding: Decode the message using the code table.

○	△	+	⊥	□	X	◇	T	⌐	=
A	B	C	D	E	F	G	H	I	J

∧	⊘	‖	<	▽	L	→	÷	\	−
K	L	M	N	O	P	Q	R	S	T

∨	←	⊠	↑	>	·¦·	↓	/	)	(
U	V	W	X	Y	Z	,	.	'	?

< ▽ ⊠ ○ ⊥ ○ > \   ‖ □ <
N O W A D A Y S   M E N

⊘ □ ○ ⊥   ⊘ ⌐ ← □ \
L E A D   L I V E S

▽ X   < ▽ ⌐ \ >
O F   N O I S Y

⊥ □ \ L □ ÷ ○ − ⌐ ▽ < /
D E S P E R A T I O N .

-- James Thurber

Time: min. ____ sec. ____

XI. Name as many TV programs as you can in one minute.

_____   _____

_____   _____

_____   _____

_____   _____

_____   _____

_____   _____

_____   _____

_____   _____

XII. Write as many of the To-Do list items as you can remember.

_____

_____

_____

_____

_____

_____

_____

XIII. Write as much as you can of the Fact of the Day.

_____

_____

_____

_____

I. Word Matrix (Find the following words in the matrix.)

1. APPLE
2. BLUEBERRY
3. CANTALOUPE
4. CHERRY
5. CRANBERRY
6. GRAPE
7. PEAR
8. RASPBERRY
9. STRAWBERRY
10. COCONUT

```
W  G  P  B  N  W  G  Q  L  Z  Z  K
E  N  Z  U  K  V  I  E  L  P  P  A
E  R  Y  Q  R  S  N  X  T  A  Y  C
P  A  Q  R  U  B  M  C  T  R  A  Y
A  S  Y  R  R  E  H  C  R  N  A  R
R  P  B  P  A  E  Q  E  T  O  L  R
G  B  M  E  B  S  B  A  Y  L  L  E
S  E  R  A  E  W  L  E  J  N  W  B
M  R  Q  R  A  O  O  F  U  D  N  N
J  R  G  R  U  K  K  M  F  L  V  A
Q  Y  T  P  X  X  D  T  D  E  B  R
W  S  E  T  U  N  O  C  O  C  I  C
```

Time: min. _____ sec. _____

II. Shopping List(Read aloud, cover, repeat aloud -- three times.)

shrimp
tomatoes
grapes
asparagus
clams
pancake syrup
butter
apricots
cream
figs

III. Fact of the Day (Read aloud, cover, and say aloud -- three times.)

As of 2002, there were 590 million passenger cars worldwide (roughly one car for every eleven people), of which 140 million were in the U.S. (roughly one car for every two people).

IV. Write as many of the Shopping List items as you can remember.

_____ _____

_____ _____

_____ _____

_____ _____

_____ _____

V. Write as much as you can of the Fact of the Day.

_____

_____

_____

_____

VI. Word Chains

start	scone	slope	flag
____	____	____	____
____	____	____	____
stone	stale	scare	____
			soar

Time: min. _____ sec. _____

VII. Coding: Decode the message using the code table.

○	△	+	⊥	□	X	◇	T	⌐	=
A	B	C	D	E	F	G	H	I	J

∧	⊘	‖	<	▽	L	→	÷	\	−
K	L	M	N	O	P	Q	R	S	T

∨	←	⊠	↑	>	⊹	↓	/	)	(
U	V	W	X	Y	Z	,	.	'	?

÷ □ L □ − ⌐ − ⌐ ▽ <   ⊥ ▽ □ \
— — — — — — — — — —   — — — —

< ▽ −   − ÷ ○ < \ X ▽ ÷ ‖   ○
— — —   — — — — — — — — —   —

⊘ ⌐ □   ⌐ < − ▽   ○
— — —   — — — —   —

− ÷ ∨ − T /
— — — — — —

-- Franklin D. Roosevelt

Time: min. _____ sec. _____

111

VIII. Schedule (You may wish to review "Calculating the Length of a Flight" on page 55 before doing part (a))

orig	dest	depart	arrive	flt#
HNL	SFO	11:00p	5:58a*	222
SFO	MSP	12:30a	5:57a	362
SFO	MSP	6:30a	12:10p	368
SFO	MSP	8:30a	2:03p	222
SFO	MSP	12:17p	5:57p	360

city	code	time
Honolulu	HNL	GMT-10
Minneapolis	MSP	GMT-6
San Francisco	SFO	GMT-8

* next day (Don't forget that "next day" may require adding 24:00)

a) What is the flying time from Honolulu to San Francisco?_____

b) Assuming that you need one hour transit time, what is the first flight you can take to Minneapolis after flying from Honolulu?_____

c) What is the time in Honolulu when you arrive in Minneapolis?_____

Time: min. _____sec._____

IX. Complete the following sequences.

1	2	7	8	13	_____
27	25	22	18	13	_____
1	3	9	27	81	_____
10	5	0	-5	-10	_____
3	6	12	24	48	_____

Time: min. _____sec._____

Brain Agility Exercises

Day 9

X. Count the number of each symbol.

```
        ∧                              ∧
              ∧                          >


         <           ∧
                 <   ∧                      <   <
         >                                  <

                        >       >
                     <   <
     >               ∧   ∧   <

       >   ∧   ∧                        <

       <                        <   ∧

       >                          ∧   ∧
```

∧ _____ < _____ > _____

Time: min. _____ sec. _____

XI. Name as many athletes as you can in one minute.

_____   _____

_____   _____

_____   _____

_____   _____

_____   _____

_____   _____

_____   _____

_____   _____

_____   _____

_____   _____

XII. Write as many of the Shopping List items as you can remember.

_____   _____

_____   _____

_____   _____

_____   _____

_____   _____

XIII. Write as much as you can of the Fact of the Day.

_____

_____

_____

_____

Brain Agility Exercises

I. Complete the following sequences.

9	2	11	2	13	_____
16	1	15	2	14	_____
1	3	11	43	171	_____
4	15	6	13	8	_____
2	6	18	54	162	_____

Time: min. _____ sec. _____

II. Shopping List(Read aloud, cover, repeat aloud -- three times.)

clams
cereal
toothpicks
pickles
honey
jelly
whole wheat flour
sugar
bananas
applesauce

III. Fact of the Day (Read aloud, cover, and say aloud -- three times.)

Internal combustion engine automobiles were first produced in Germany by Karl Benz in 1885-1886 and Gottlieb Daimler between 1886-1889.

IV. Write as many of the Shopping List items as you can remember.

_____   _____

_____   _____

_____   _____

_____   _____

_____   _____

V. Write as much as you can of the Fact of the Day.

_____

_____

_____

_____

VI. Word Chains

find	calf	blow	sold
____	____	____	____
____	____	____	____
land	bawl	boat	____
			bill

Time: min. _____ sec. _____

VII. Find the figures which are rotations and not reflections of the figure at the left of each line.

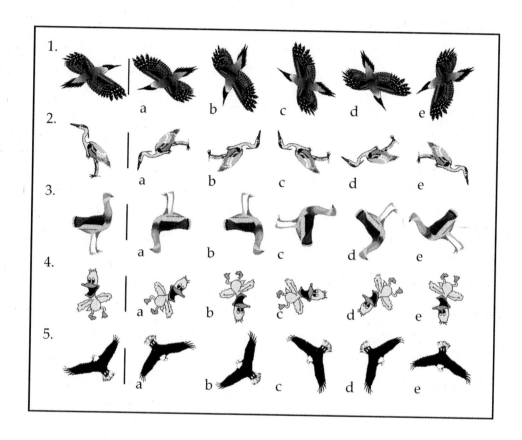

1)_____ 2)_____ 3)_____ 4)_____ 5)_____

Time: min. ____ sec. ____

VIII. Calculate the following:

58105	68113	22637	21126	86127
23680	17432	46863	37126	18978

22663	47318	86770	34933	14160
75746	28332	71120	51650	11301

Time: min. _____sec._____

IX. Find as many words of three letters or more which can be made from the letters of the following word. (Time limit - 3 minutes)

AMERICA

_____   _____

_____   _____

_____   _____

_____   _____

_____   _____

_____   _____

_____   _____

X. Count the number of each symbol.

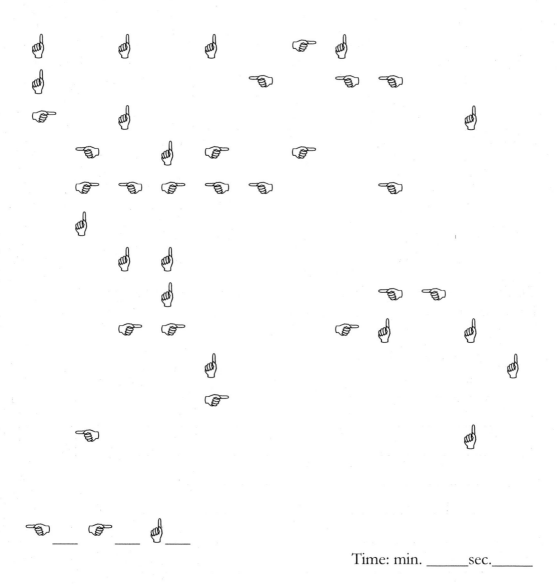

Time: min. _____ sec. _____

XI. Name as many vegetables as you can in one minute.

_____	_____
_____	_____
_____	_____
_____	_____
_____	_____
_____	_____
_____	_____
_____	_____
_____	_____
_____	_____

XII. Write as many of the Shopping List items as you can remember.

_____	_____
_____	_____
_____	_____
_____	_____
_____	_____

XIII. Write as much as you can of the Fact of the Day.

_____

_____

_____

_____

I. Word Matrix (Find the following words in the matrix.)

I	L	G	U	I	E	N	G	L	A	N	D
S	W	I	T	Z	E	R	L	A	N	D	S
V	B	W	J	K	R	A	M	N	E	D	A
E	R	J	X	A	N	K	N	V	W	N	X
Z	A	A	G	R	C	A	T	R	G	G	F
S	Z	P	I	G	J	H	N	E	N	N	X
X	I	A	R	E	M	N	I	I	B	H	H
N	L	N	C	N	M	E	Z	L	H	I	X
J	Q	D	I	T	I	Y	X	W	E	C	T
A	U	I	W	I	J	L	Z	I	Q	T	G
Z	I	C	K	N	Z	S	I	P	C	S	E
X	S	B	A	A	O	E	Y	O	L	O	P

1. Argentina
2. Brazil
3. Chile
4. Denmark
5. England
6. Japan
7. Mexico
8. Switzerland
9. Tibet
10. China

Time: min. _____ sec. _____

II. To-Do List(Read aloud, cover, repeat aloud -- three times.)

do brain agility exercises
get haircut
reconcile bank statement
have tires rotated
have photos printed
put gas in car
call computer repair

III. Fact of the Day (Read aloud, cover, and say aloud -- three times.)

The United States is the largest exporter of weapons in the world, with military sales constituting about 18 percent of the GNP, the greatest proportion of any nation.

IV. Write as many of the To-Do list items as you can remember.

_____

_____

_____

_____

_____

_____

_____

V. Write as much as you can of the Fact of the Day.

_____

_____

_____

_____

_____

VI. Schedule

orig	dest	depart	arrive	flt#	city	code	time
AMS	DTW	8:00a	10:55a	39	Amsterdam	AMS	GMT+1
AMS	DTW	10:50a	1:45p	67	Bombay	BOM	GMT+5.5
AMS	DTW	3:40p	6:35p	53	Detroit	DTW	GMT-5
BOM	AMS	1:20a	6:45a	33			

a) How long is flight 39 from Amsterdam to Detroit?_____

b) When you arrive in Detroit on flight 39, what is the time in Bombay?_____

Time: min. _____sec._____

VII. Find the figures which are rotations and not reflections of the figure at the left of each line.

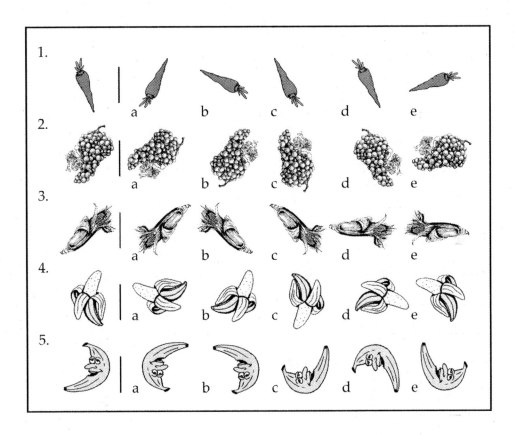

1)_____ 2)_____ 3)_____ 4)_____ 5)_____

Time: min. ____ sec. ____

VIII. Calculate the following:

90220	64065	68268	36690	44806
84318	39211	98089	98566	51807

98361	54081	76337	65531	99423
-69534	-36243	-67734	-28990	-42666

Time: min. _____sec._____

IX. Find as many words of four letters or more which can be made from the letters of the following word. (Time limit - 3 minutes)

HOPEFUL

_____   _____

_____   _____

_____   _____

_____   _____

_____   _____

_____   _____

_____   _____

X. Coding: Decode the message using the code table.

○	△	+	⊥	□	X	◇	T	⌐	=
A	B	C	D	E	F	G	H	I	J

∧	⊘	‖	<	▽	L	→	÷	\	—
K	L	M	N	O	P	Q	R	S	T

∨	←	⊠	↑	>	·ǀ·	↓	/	`	)	(
U	V	W	X	Y	Z	,	.	`	`	?

+ ○ ⊘ ⌐ X ▽ ÷ < ⌐ ○   ⌐ \   ○
— — — — — — — — —   — —   —

X ⌐ < □   L ⊘ ○ + □   — ▽
— — — —   — — — — —   — —

⊘ ⌐ ← □ ↓   ⌐ X   > ▽ ∨
— — — — —   — —   — — —

T ○ L L □ <   — ▽   △ □   ○ <
— — — — — —   — —   — —   — —

▽ ÷ ○ < ◇ □ /
— — — — — — —

-- Fred Allen

Time: min. _____ sec. _____

XI. Name as many fruits as you can in one minute.

_____   _____

_____   _____

_____   _____

_____   _____

_____   _____

_____   _____

_____   _____

_____   _____

XII. Write as many of the To-Do list items as you can remember.

_____

_____

_____

_____

_____

_____

_____

XIII. Write as much as you can of the Fact of the Day.

_____

_____

_____

_____

I. Word Matrix (Find the following words in the matrix.)

```
 1. FORSYTHIA
 2. LILY
 3. LOBELIA
 4. MARIGOLD
 5. PERIWINKLE
 6. RHODODENDRON
 7. ROSE
 8. TULIP
 9. ZINNIA
10. FLOX
```

```
M F G D G R A F T U G L
V P O V L I L Z T T I P
U W J R L O E N J L L E
H J G E S W G S Y E Y R
K T B B I Y A I O F X I
U O D Y O I T X R R Z W
L T O Y N N S H B A R I
A E U N Z X G X I P M N
E K I L N V O W C A T K
P Z K Q I L C I W Y X L
L M Y U F P B J S Z U E
R H O D O D E N D R O N
```

Time: min. _____ sec. _____

II. Shopping List(Read aloud, cover, repeat aloud -- three times.)

milk
green onions
applesauce
garlic
dog food
beets
watermelon
salt
catsup
soup

III. Fact of the Day (Read aloud, cover, and say aloud -- three times.)

Wikipedia, a web-based, free-content, encyclopedia project started in 2001, has grown to over six million articles in 250 languages, including 1.6 million in the English-language edition.

IV. Write as many of the Shopping List items as you can remember.

_____	_____
_____	_____
_____	_____
_____	_____
_____	_____

V. Write as much as you can of the Fact of the Day.

_____

_____

_____

_____

VI. Word Chains

blow	snip	coal	trade
____	____	____	____
____	____	____	____
flag	flap	gold	____
			blame

Time: min. _____ sec. _____

Brain Agility Exercises

VII. Coding: Decode the message using the code table.

○	△	+	⊥	□	X	◇	T	⌐	=
A	B	C	D	E	F	G	H	I	J

∧	⊘	‖	<	▽	L	→	÷	\	−
K	L	M	N	O	P	Q	R	S	T

∨	←	⊠	↑	>	⊹	↓	/	)	(
U	V	W	X	Y	Z	,	.	'	?

\ ⌐ ⊘ □ < + □   ⌐ \
— — — — — — —   — —
S I L E N C E   I S

◇ ▽ ⊘ ⊥ □ <   ⊠ T □ <
— — — — — —   — — — —
G O L D E N   W H E N

> ▽ ∨   + ○ <) −
— — —   — — — — —
Y O U   C A N ' T

− T ⌐ < ∧   ▽ X   ○
— — — — —   — —   —
T H I N K   O F   A

◇ ▽ ▽ ⊥   ○ < \ ⊠ □ ÷ /
— — — —   — — — — — — —
G O O D   A N S W E R .

-- Muhammad Ali

Time: min. _____ sec. _____

VIII. Schedule

orig	dest	depart	arrive	flt#	city	code	time
SFO	MSP	12:30a	5:57a	362	London	LGW	GMT+0
SFO	MSP	6:30a	12:10p	368	Minneapolis	MSP	GMT-6
SFO	MSP	8:30a	2:03p	222	San Francisco	SFO	GMT-8
MSP	LGW	6:50p	9:00a*	44	*next day		

a) What is the shortest overall travel time from San Francisco to

London?_____

b) How long is the flight from Minneapolis to London?_____

c) When you arrive in London, what time is it in San Francisco?_____

Time: min. _____sec._____

IX. Complete the following sequences.

6	3	18	3	54	_____
18	16	22	20	26	_____
1234	2341	3412	4123	1234	_____
2	2	3	3	3	_____
1	3	7	15	31	_____

Time: min. _____sec._____

X. Count the number of each symbol.

😊   😊   ☹   😊

😊   ☹

😐   ☹

😐   😐

😊   😊   😐   😐

☹   😊   ☹

😐   😊

☹   ☹

😐

😊   ☹   😊

😐   😊   😐

😐   😊

😊 ___   😐 ___   ☹ ___

Time: min. _____ sec. _____

XI. Name as many items of furniture as you can in one minute.

_____	_____
_____	_____
_____	_____
_____	_____
_____	_____
_____	_____
_____	_____
_____	_____
_____	_____

XII. Write as many of the Shopping List items as you can remember.

_____	_____
_____	_____
_____	_____
_____	_____
_____	_____

XIII. Write as much as you can of the Fact of the Day.

_____

_____

_____

_____

_____

Brain Agility Exercises

I. Complete the following sequences.

1	2	6	24	120	_____
100	110	111	200	220	_____
1	12	312	3124	53124	_____
3	13	22	30	37	_____
521	511	502	494	487	_____

Time: min. _____ sec._____

II. Shopping List(Read, cover, repeat aloud -- three times.)

chicken
plums
bread
prunes
figs
bacon
oranges
pasta
potato chips

III. Fact of the Day (Read aloud, cover, and say aloud -- three times.)

The share of the U.S. population age 65 and older grew from 9.5% in 1967 to 12.4% in 2005. By 2030 almost 20% of the population will be 65 or older.

IV. Write as many of the Shopping List items as you can remember.

_____   _____

_____   _____

_____   _____

_____   _____

_____   _____

V. Write as much as you can of the Fact of the Day.

_____

_____

_____

_____

VI. Word Chains

yell   head   toll   frog

_____   _____   _____   _____

_____   _____   _____   _____

call   hair   road   _____

                                    _____

                                    skip

Time: min. _____ sec. _____

Brain Agility Exercises

VII. Find the figures which are rotations and not reflections of the figure
at the left of each line.

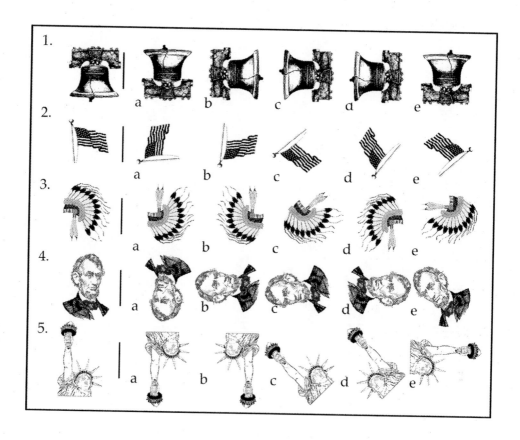

1)_____ 2)_____ 3)_____ 4)_____ 5)_____

Time: min. ____ sec. ____

VIII. Calculate the following:

63554	59386	43587	42777	61443
36176	21306	83368	87180	47293

30780	81689	96816	40713	91857
-20526	-79779	-87882	-35328	-60818

Time: min. ____ sec. ____

IX. Find as many words of three letters or more which can be made from the letters of the following word. (Time limit - 3 minutes)

LAUGHTER

_____   _____

_____   _____

_____   _____

_____   _____

_____   _____

_____   _____

_____   _____

X. Count the number of each symbol.

↗ ↙

↘   ↗ ↙   ↙   ↙

↗ ↙

↗   ↘

↘ ↘

↗   ↙

↙   ↘

↙   ↘

↙   ↗   ↗   ↗

↗   ↘   ↘   ↙ ↘

↗____   ↙____   ↘____

Time: min. _____sec._____

XI. Name as many birds as you can in one minute.

_____   _____

_____   _____

_____   _____

_____   _____

_____   _____

_____   _____

_____   _____

_____   _____

_____   _____

XII. Write as many of the Shopping List items as you can remember.

_____   _____

_____   _____

_____   _____

_____   _____

_____   _____

XIII. Write as much as you can of the Fact of the Day.

_____

_____

_____

_____

I. Word Matrix (Find the following words in the matrix.)

1. CALIFORNIA
2. DELAWARE
3. FLORIDA
4. IOWA
5. MARYLAND
6. MINNESOTA
7. MISSOURI
8. NEVADA
9. PENNSYLVANIA
10. RHODE ISLAND

```
I A E U W J X C D S X F
R C I N E V A D A Y M M
U T W N V H E S A S A T
O J Y S R L K T B D R I
S D O W A O O X I Y Y H
S H Y W S S F R R Q L I
I J A Y E O O I R T A O
M R A N M L O O L U N W
E W N X F G T J H A D A
L I K N V V Q Z Z L C S
M D N A L S I E D O H R
A I N A V L Y S N N E P
```

Time: min. ____ sec. ____

II. To-Do List(Read aloud, cover, repeat aloud -- three times.)

call travel agent
renew newspaper
renew prescription
buy concert tickets
doctor's appointment
write letter to congressional reps
water plants

III. Fact of the Day (Read aloud, cover, and say aloud -- three times.)

The United Nations, founded in 1945, has 192 member states. On January 1, 2007 Ban Ki-moon became the Secretary-General of the U.N.

IV. Write as many of the To-Do list items as you can remember.

_____

_____

_____

_____

_____

_____

_____

V. Write as much as you can of the Fact of the Day.

_____

_____

_____

_____

VI. Schedule

orig	dest	depart	arrive	flt#	city	code	time
AMS	BOM	10:10a	11:20p	34	Amsterdam	AMS	GMT+1
MSP	AMS	3:20p	6:30a*	42	Bombay	BOM	GMT+5.5
MSP	AMS	9:20p	12:40p*	56	Minneapolis	MSP	GMT-6
SFO	MSP	12:30a	5:57a	362	San Francisco	SFO	GMT-8
SFO	MSP	6:30a	12:10p	368	* next day		
SFO	MSP	8:30a	2:03p	222			

a) What is the latest time you can leave San Francisco for Bombay?_____

c) How long is flight 42 from Minneapolis to Amsterdam ?_____

d) When you arrive in Amsterdam, what time is it in San Francisco?_____

Time: min. _____sec._____

VII. Find the figures which are rotations and not reflections of the figure at the left of each line.

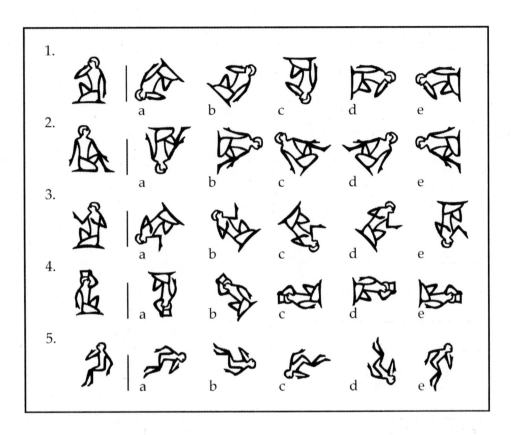

1)_____ 2)_____ 3)_____ 4)_____ 5)_____

Time: min. _____sec._____

VIII. Calculate the following:

38637	96898	60069	57823	56086
16872	14241	84297	87208	86513

66039	33687	75584	88633	96843
-56972	-28814	-34409	-18756	-85939

Time: min. _____sec._____

IX. Find as many words of three letters or more which can be made from the letters of the following word. (Time limit - 3 minutes)

INFORMATION

_____	_____
_____	_____
_____	_____
_____	_____
_____	_____
_____	_____
_____	_____

Brain Agility Exercises

X. Coding: Decode the message using the code table.

○	△	+	⊥	□	X	◇	T	⌐	=
A	B	C	D	E	F	G	H	I	J

∧	⊘	‖	<	▽	L	→	÷	\	—
K	L	M	N	O	P	Q	R	S	T

V	⇐	⊠	↑	>	·⊦	↓	/	`	⊂
U	V	W	X	Y	Z	,	.	`	?

⊠ T □ <   > ▽ V   ◇ □ —
_ _ _ _   _ _ _   _ _ _

— ▽   — T □   □ < ⊥   ▽ X
_ _   _ _ _   _ _ _   _ _

> ▽ V ÷   ÷ ▽ L □ ↓
_ _ _ _   _ _ _ _ _

— ⌐ □   ○   ∧ < ▽ —
_ _ _   _   _ _ _ _

○ < ⊥   T ○ < ◇   ▽ < /
_ _ _   _ _ _ _   _ _ _

-- Franklin D. Roosevelt

Time: min. ____ sec. ____

143

XI. Name as many colors as you can in one minute.

_____   _____

_____   _____

_____   _____

_____   _____

_____   _____

_____   _____

_____   _____

_____   _____

XII. Write as many of the To-Do list items as you can remember.

_____

_____

_____

_____

_____

_____

_____

XIII. Write as much as you can of the Fact of the Day.

_____

_____

_____

_____

I. Word Matrix (Find the following words in the matrix.)

1. BABOON
2. GORILLA
3. LEMUR
4. LEOPARD
5. LION
6. PANTHER
7. SLOTH
8. TIGER
9. ZEBRA
10. DEER

```
V R J W R W A A B X U A
R W U I Q A X A F D F Q
E G W M Z R B K N A Z G
G S S E E O E Z M X Q Z
I A B S O L T E P C A K
T R L N W U O O D B F E
A X U L D L B L I I E J
X N T Z I R E A J E A Y
L Q D I F R P C N M B H
S L O T H S O Y U O O L
D R A P O E L G Z I I G
W K N J P A N T H E R L
```

Time: min. ____ sec. ____

II. Shopping List(Read aloud, cover, repeat aloud -- three times.)

lettuce
soup
eggs
onions
laundry detergent
carrots
peaches
mushrooms
trout
ice cream

III. Fact of the Day (Read aloud, cover, and say aloud -- three times.)

The moon is about one-third the size of the earth and is about 238,000 miles from the earth.

IV. Write as many of the Shopping List items as you can remember.

_____	_____
_____	_____
_____	_____
_____	_____
_____	_____

V. Write as much as you can of the Fact of the Day.

_____

_____

_____

_____

VI. Word Chains

game	bawl	heat	bald
____	____	____	____
____	____	____	____
tale	yell	____	____
		cold	hair

Time: min. ____ sec. ____

Brain Agility Exercises

VII. Coding: Decode the message using the code table.

○	△	+	⊥	□	×	◇	T	⌐	=
A	B	C	D	E	F	G	H	I	J

∧	⊘	‖	<	▽	L	→	÷	\	—
K	L	M	N	O	P	Q	R	S	T

∨	←	⊠	↑	>	·|·	↓	/	)	(
U	V	W	X	Y	Z	,	.	'	?

○ ◇ □   ⌐ \   ○
‾ ‾ ‾   ‾ ‾   ‾

→ ∨ □ \ — ⌐ ▽ <   ▽ ×
‾ ‾ ‾ ‾ ‾ ‾ ‾ ‾   ‾ ‾

‖ ⌐ < ⊥   ▽ ← □ ÷
‾ ‾ ‾ ‾   ‾ ‾ ‾ ‾

‖ ○ — — □ ÷ /   ⌐ ×   > ▽ ∨
‾ ‾ ‾ ‾ ‾ ‾ ‾   ‾ ‾   ‾ ‾ ‾

⊥ ▽ <) —   ‖ ⌐ < ⊥ ↓   ⌐ —
‾ ‾ ‾ ‾ ‾   ‾ ‾ ‾ ‾ ‾   ‾ ‾

⊥ ▽ □ \ <) —   ‖ ○ — — □ ÷
‾ ‾ ‾ ‾ ‾ ‾ ‾   ‾ ‾ ‾ ‾ ‾ ‾

-- Satchel Paige

Time: min. _____ sec. _____

147

VIII. Schedule

orig	dest	depart	arrive	flt#
BOS	DTW	6:00a	8:15a	371
BOS	DTW	7:06a	9:23a	377
BOS	DTW	9:04a	11:25a	375
BOS	DTW	11:59a	2:14p	1195
BOS	DTW	2:37p	4:54p	381
BOS	DTW	4:12p	6:29p	207
BOS	DTW	5:48p	8:08p	373
BOS	DTW	7:37p	9:49p	379
DTW	SFO	9:22a	11:25a	343
DTW	SFO	12:15p	2:22p	345
DTW	SFO	7:39p	9:51p	347
SFO	NRT	12:00p	4:30p*	27

city	code	time
Boston	BOS	GMT-5
Detroit	DTW	GMT-5
San Francisco	SFO	GMT-8
Tokyo	NRT	GMT+9

* next day

a) If you need at least 30 minutes transit time, what is the latest time you can
   leave Boston for Tokyo?_____

b) How long is the flight from San Francisco to Tokyo?_____

c) When you arrive in Tokyo, what time is it in Boston?_____

Time: min. _____sec._____

IX. Complete the following sequences.

9	4	14	4	19	_____
200	136	104	88	80	_____
1	21	213	4213	42135	_____
4	2	9	2	14	_____
63	57	52	47	43	_____

Time: min. _____sec._____

X. Count the number of each symbol.

△___ ▽___ ◁___ ▷___

Time: min. _____ sec. _____

XI. Name as many items of clothing as you can in one minute.

_____   _____

_____   _____

_____   _____

_____   _____

_____   _____

_____   _____

_____   _____

_____   _____

_____   _____

_____   _____

XII. Write as many of the Shopping List items as you can remember.

_____   _____

_____   _____

_____   _____

_____   _____

_____   _____

XIII. Write as much as you can of the Fact of the Day.

_____

_____

_____

_____

Brain Agility Exercises   Day 16

I. Complete the following sequences.

5	13	7	16	9	_____
35	5	30	10	25	_____
2573	3257	4325	5432	6543	_____
2	3	5	9	17	_____
3	7	16	32	57	_____

Time: min. _____sec._____

II. Shopping List(Read aloud, cover, repeat aloud -- three times.)

spaghetti
tomato soup
toothpaste
pot roast
eggs
ice cream
flour
paper napkins
green beans

III. Fact of the Day (Read aloud, cover, and say aloud -- three times.)

Oceans cover almost three-quarters of the earth's surface, with almost half of the water over 9,000 feet deep.

IV. Write as many of the Shopping List items as you can remember.

_____   _____

_____   _____

_____   _____

_____   _____

_____   _____

V. Write as much as you can of the Fact of the Day.

_____

_____

_____

_____

VI. Word Chains

sport   stow

_____   _____

_____   _____

_____   _____

stars   _____

                         boat

Time: min. ____ sec. ____

VII. Find the figures which are rotations and not reflections of the figure
     at the left of each line.

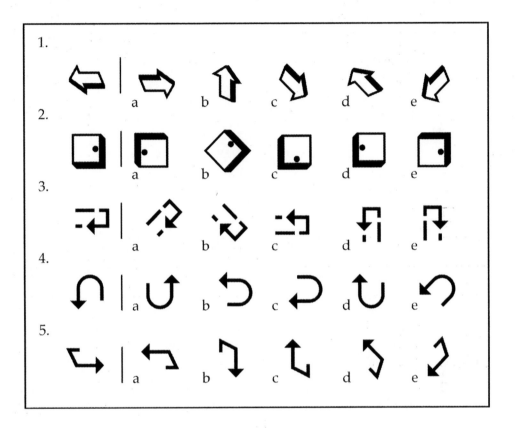

1)_____ 2)_____ 3)_____ 4)_____ 5)_____

Time: min. ____ sec. ____

VIII. Calculate the following:

86938	90598	11547	56776	79242
31208	94378	48286	68485	27926

44953	73200	97464	51827	86397
-26704	-49203	-95027	-27263	-57264

Time: min. ____ sec. ____

IX. Find as many words of three letters or more which can be made from the letters of the following word. (Time limit - 3 minutes)

SUNSHINE

_____	_____
_____	_____
_____	_____
_____	_____
_____	_____
_____	_____
_____	_____

X. Count the number of each symbol.

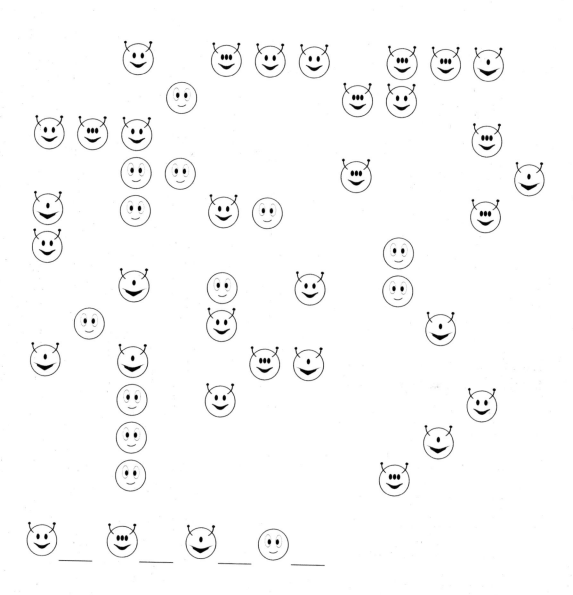

Time: min. _____ sec. _____

XI. Name as many emotions as you can in one minute.

_____	_____
_____	_____
_____	_____
_____	_____
_____	_____
_____	_____
_____	_____
_____	_____
_____	_____
_____	_____

XII. Write as many of the Shopping List items as you can remember.

_____	_____
_____	_____
_____	_____
_____	_____
_____	_____

XIII. Write as much as you can of the Fact of the Day.

_____

_____

_____

_____

I. Word Matrix (Find the following words in the matrix.)

1. BASSOON
2. CLARINET
3. FLUTE
4. FRENCH HORN
5. OBOE
6. ORGAN
7. PIANO
8. TROMBONE
9. TRUMPET
10. VIOLA

```
N V O P C L N P Y Q Q O
F X I F G B A S S O O N
W R T O J D Q A T S T O
T C E R L S Z M T F B N
E L L N O A M E V O P O
P M P A C M K W E F O N
M O O J R H B C Z L N A
U X N F Z I H O X U J I
R X Z K O T N O N T V P
T D S V R Y M E R E M I
L T M Q H P Z F T N F I
X S Y J X K O R G A N M
```

Time: min. _____ sec. _____

II. To-Do List(Read aloud, cover, repeat aloud -- three times.)

buy theater tickets
make jam for county fair
fertilize rhododendrons
recycle newspapers
make appointment for eye exam
have tires on car rotated
clean aquarium filter

III. Fact of the Day (Read aloud, cover, and say aloud -- three times.)

In 1948 Costa Rica abolished its military and dedicated the former military budget to education, culture, and security.

IV. Write as many of the To-Do list items as you can remember.

_____

_____

_____

_____

_____

_____

_____

V. Write as much as you can of the Fact of the Day.

_____

_____

_____

_____

VI. Schedule

orig	dest	depart	arrive	flt#	city	code	time
JFK	DTW	9:02a	11:13a	898	New York	JFK	GMT-5
JFK	DTW	12:35p	2:53p	894	Detroit	DTW	GMT-5
JFK	DTW	4:11p	6:25p	896	Tokyo	NRT	GMT+9
DTW	NRT	12:35p	4:00*p	11			
DTW	NRT	1:40p	5:05p*	25	*next day		

a) What is the latest you can leave New York for Tokyo without staying overnight in Detroit?_____

b) What is the flying time on flight 25 to Tokyo?_____

c) What time is it in New York when arriving in Tokyo on flight 25?_____

Time: min. _____sec._____

VII. Find the figures which are rotations and not reflections of the figure at the left of each line.

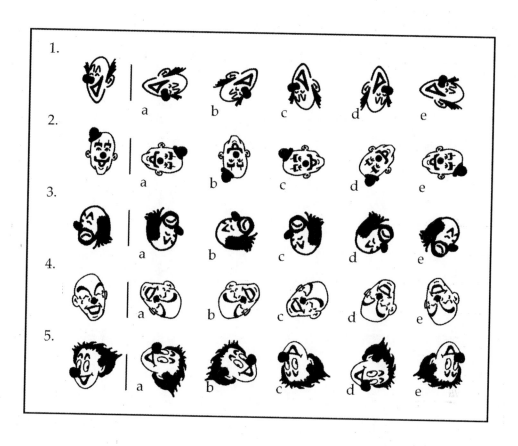

1) _____ 2) _____ 3) _____ 4) _____ 5) _____

Time: min. _____ sec. _____

VIII. Calculate the following:

44593	9100	68320	95014	30461
38069	15065	54033	52525	53542

85574	74963	95334	82206	93600
-65772	-58412	-80594	-76576	-74027

Time: min. _____sec._____

IX. Find as many words of three letters or more which can be made from the letters of the following word. (Time limit - 3 minutes)

SEATTLE

_____   _____

_____   _____

_____   _____

_____   _____

_____   _____

_____   _____

_____   _____

X. Coding: Decode the message using the code table.

⇨	⇦	⇨	⇦	⇨	←	→	↑	↓	↖
A	B	C	D	E	F	G	H	I	J

↗	↙	↘	↔	↕	▲	▼	△	▽	◀
K	L	M	N	O	P	Q	R	S	T

▶	◁	▷	◣	◤	◢	⊥	↘	⇦	⌐
U	V	W	X	Y	Z	,	.	'	?

▷ ↑ ⇨ ↔   ◀ ↑ ⇨   ⇨ ⇨ → ↙ ⇨ ▽

_ _ _ _   _ _ _   _ _ _ _ _ _

⇨ △ ⇨   ▽ ↓ ↙ ⇨ ↔ ◀ ⊥   ◀ ↑ ⇨

_ _ _   _ _ _ _ _ _ _   _ _ _

▲ ⇨ △ △ ↕ ◀ ▽   ⇦ ⇨ → ↓ ↔

_ _ _ _ _ _ _   _ _ _ _ _

◀ ↕   ↖ ⇨ ⇦ ⇦ ⇨ △ ↘

_ _   _ _ _ _ _ _ _

-- Winston Churchill

Time: min. ____ sec. ____

XI. Name as many animals that live in the water as you can in one minute.

_____   _____

_____   _____

_____   _____

_____   _____

_____   _____

_____   _____

_____   _____

_____   _____

XII. Write as many of the To-Do list items as you can remember.

_____

_____

_____

_____

_____

_____

_____

XIII. Write as much as you can of the Fact of the Day.

_____

_____

_____

_____

I. Word Matrix (Find the following words in the matrix.)

1.	CANARY
2.	CAT
3.	DOG
4.	FERRET
5.	GUINEA PIG
6.	HAMSTER
7.	MONKEY
8.	PARAKEET
9.	PARROT
10.	TURTLE

```
Y N F P K H A M S T E R
V E F R O D B Z A P D Z
G K K T K T C A K G C B
V M B N U Z I O I I E O
Y G P R O C F P P M E Z
I R T A Q M A E A M E K
R L A Y R E U T R G B I
E U W N N A M L R R Q T
V T B I A F K D O G E R
K I U W G C E E T U C T
M G O H I E X Q E T V N
D P U F L F P X Q T H M
```

Time: min. ____ sec. ____

II. Shopping List(Read aloud, cover, repeat aloud -- three times.)

sugar
beets
tea
swiss chard
grapefruit
yogurt
green onions
apples
eggplant
salmon

III. Fact of the Day (Read aloud, cover, and say aloud -- three times.)

Although Alexander Fleming discovered penicillin in 1928, it was not until 1942 that John Bumstead and Orvan Hess successfully used it to treat human infection.

IV. Write as many of the Shopping List items as you can remember.

_____   _____

_____   _____

_____   _____

_____   _____

_____   _____

V. Write as much as you can of the Fact of the Day.

_____

_____

_____

_____

VI. Word Chains

plant   loot

_____   _____

_____   _____

_____   _____

_____   _____

stars   gold

Time: min. ____ sec. ____

Brain Agility Exercises

VII. Coding: Decode the message using the code table.

○	△	+	⊥	□	✗	◇	T	⅃	=
A	B	C	D	E	F	G	H	I	J

∧	⊘	‖	<	▽	L	→	÷	\	—
K	L	M	N	O	P	Q	R	S	T

∨	←	⊠	↑	>	·⊦	↓	/	)	(
U	V	W	X	Y	Z	,	.	'	?

⅃ —   ⅃ \   △ □ — — □ ÷   — ▽

__ __   __ __   __ __ __ __ __ __   __ __

∧ < ▽ ⊠   \ ▽ ‖ □   ▽ ✗

__ __ __ __   __ __ __ __   __ __

— T □   → ∨ □ \ — ⅃ ▽ < \

__ __ __   __ __ __ __ __ __ __ __ __

— T ○ <   ○ ⊘ ⊘   ▽ ✗   — T □

__ __ __ __   __ __ __   __ __   __ __ __

○ < \ ⊠ □ ÷ \ /

__ __ __ __ __ __ __ __

-- James Thurber

Time: min. _____ sec._____

165

VIII. Schedule

orig	dest	depart	arrive	flt#
DTW	NRT	12:35p	4:00*p	11
DTW	NRT	1:40p	5:05p*	25
MIA	DTW	7:50a	10:59a	992
MIA	DTW	1:24p	4:28p	986
MIA	DTW	2:40p	5:48p	996
NRT	BKK	6:25p	11:55p	27

city	code	time
Bangkok	BKK	GMT+7
Detroit	DTW	GMT-5
Miami	MIA	GMT-5
Tokyo	NRT	GMT+9

* next day

a) What is the latest time you can leave Miami to fly to Bangkok?_____

b) What is the total travel time to Bangkok?_____

c) When you arrive in Bangkok, what time is it in Miami?_____

Time: min. _____sec._____

IX. Complete the following sequences.

09   81   27   63   45   _____

29   A   25   B   21   _____

2   4   6   10   16   _____

C   E   G   I   K   _____

2   5   11   23   47   _____

Time: min. _____sec._____

Brain Agility Exercises

X. Count the number of each symbol.

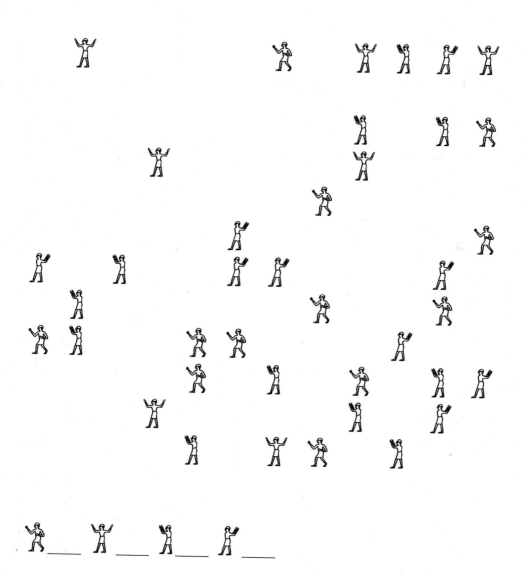

XI. Name as many virtues as you can in one minute.

_____	_____
_____	_____
_____	_____
_____	_____
_____	_____
_____	_____
_____	_____
_____	_____
_____	_____
_____	_____

XII. Write as many of the Shopping List items as you can remember.

_____	_____
_____	_____
_____	_____
_____	_____
_____	_____

XIII. Write as much as you can of the Fact of the Day.

_____

_____

_____

_____

I. Complete the following sequences.

7	5	12	17	29	_____
29	23	28	24	27	_____
4	6	10	18	34	_____
D	G	J	M	P	_____
1928374	147382	12837	1738	183	_____

Time: min. _____sec._____

II. Shopping List(Read aloud, cover, repeat aloud -- three times.)

broccoli
olive oil
cabbage
squash
vinegar
flour
potatoes
minestrone
applesauce
peaches

III. Fact of the Day (Read aloud, cover, and say aloud -- three times.)

The Blue Whale, a marine mammal at up to 110 feet in length and 200 tons in weight, is believed to be the largest animal to have ever lived on Earth though some recent dinosaur discoveries may contradict this long-held belief.

IV. Write as many of the Shopping List items as you can remember.

_____   _____

_____   _____

_____   _____

_____   _____

_____   _____

V. Write as much as you can of the Fact of the Day.

_____

_____

_____

_____

VI. Word Chains

snow   blow

_____   _____

_____   _____

_____   _____

_____   _____

coat   cold

Time: min. ____ sec. ____

170

Brain Agility Exercises

VII. Find the figures which are rotations and not reflections of the figure
at the left of each line.

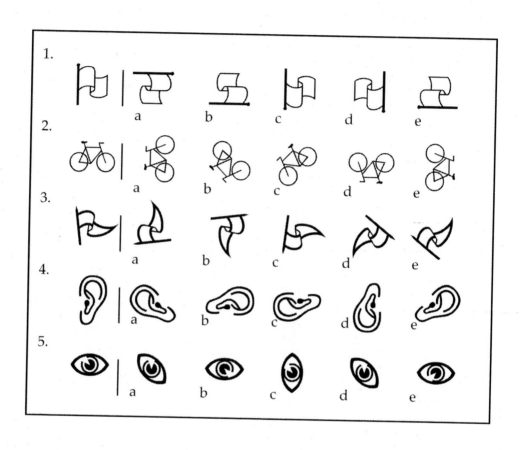

1)_____ 2)_____ 3)_____ 4)_____ 5)_____

Time: min. ____ sec. ____

VIII. Calculate the following:

56791	81023	37645	82002	34255
64466	92038	28973	12551	99657

88431	94099	88885	98867	73591
-81401	-89661	-57573	-68223	-36677

Time: min. ____ sec. ____

IX. Find as many words of three letters or more which can be made from the letters of the following word. (Time limit - 3 minutes)

AIRPLANE

_____   _____

_____   _____

_____   _____

_____   _____

_____   _____

_____   _____

_____   _____

Brain Agility Exercises

X. Count the number of each symbol.

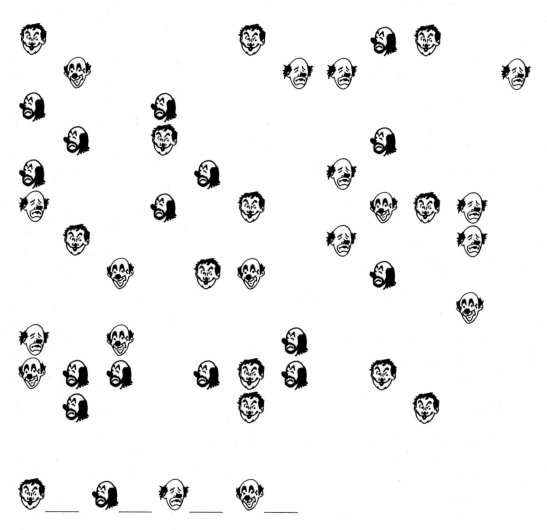

Time: min. _____sec._____

XI. Name as many occupations as you can in one minute.

_____   _____
_____   _____
_____   _____
_____   _____
_____   _____
_____   _____
_____   _____
_____   _____
_____   _____
_____   _____

XII. Write as many of the Shopping List items as you can remember.

_____   _____
_____   _____
_____   _____
_____   _____
_____   _____

XIII. Write as much as you can of the Fact of the Day.

_____
_____
_____
_____

I. Word Matrix (Find the following words in the matrix.)

1. APPLES
2. BREAD
3. BUTTER
4. CELERY
5. MACARONI
6. MILK
7. NOODLES
8. PORK
9. RICE
10. CHEESE

```
N P Y I A L R I U B K N
O K K A I H N C M I G P
O B R Q P O C K B O F K
D V G O R P B R E A D P
L K L A P F L Z K O P I
E J C X Y K U E M I L K
S A E U R H M K S R D C
M M C U E O U B E Y H D
F I I U L B G T S E Y Q
F Q R C E K T W E U H L
J I G K C U J S L B S I
Q F L M B R E J D L J W
```

Time: min. ____ sec. ____

II. To-Do List(Read aloud, cover, repeat aloud -- three times.)

take car in for repair
renew prescription
have photos printed
do brain agility exercises
dental appointment
put gas in car
write letter to congressional reps

III. Fact of the Day (Read aloud, cover, and say aloud -- three times.)

At the end of 2006, the world's population reached 6.5 billion. The
two largest populations are in China (1.3 billion) and India (1.1
billion). The population of the United States is just over 300 million.

IV. Write as many of the To-Do list items as you can remember.

_____

_____

_____

_____

_____

_____

_____

V. Write as much as you can of the Fact of the Day.

_____

_____

_____

_____

VI. Schedule

orig	dest	depart	arrive	flt#	city	code	time
AMS	MSP	10:10a	12:20p	41	Amsterdam	AMS	GMT+1
AMS	MSP	1:15p	3:20p	45	Bombay	BOM	GMT+5.5
BOM	AMS	1:20a	6:45a	33	Honolulu	HNL	GMT-10
MSP	SFO	11:43a	1:46p	221	Minneapolis	MSP	GMT-6
MSP	SFO	2:40p	4:38p	369	San Francisco	SFO	GMT-8
MSP	SFO	5:22p	7:21p	357			
MSP	SFO	9:10p	11:06p	355			
SFO	HNL	3:10p	6:41p	221			

a) What is the total travel time from Bombay to Minneapolis?_____

b) Assuming you stay in Minneapolis overnight, what is the latest time you must leave Minneapolis for Honolulu?_____

c) What is the time in Amsterdam when you arrive in Honolulu?_____

Time: min. _____sec._____

VII. Find the figures which are rotations and not reflections of the figure at the left of each line.

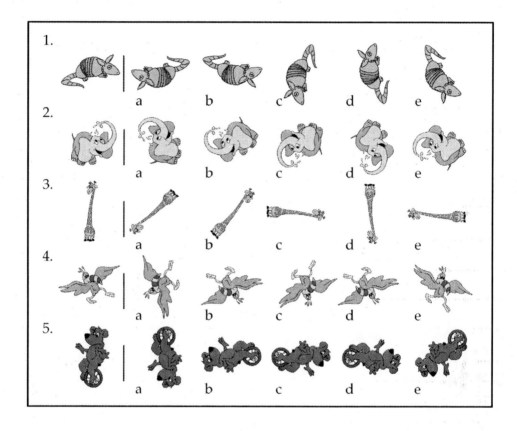

1).............. 2)............... 3)............... 4............... 5...............

Time: min. _____sec._____

VIII. Calculate the following:

97106	71683	77337	85019	73077
42292	93957	65904	52905	71877

61898	47093	88963	76391	39902
-40427	-17100	-77826	-71307	-28750

Time: min. _____ sec. _____

IX. Find as many words of three letters or more which can be made from the letters of the following word. (Time limit - 3 minutes)

SCRABBLE

_____   _____

_____   _____

_____   _____

_____   _____

_____   _____

_____   _____

_____   _____

Brain Agility Exercises

Day 20

X. Coding: Decode the message using the code table.

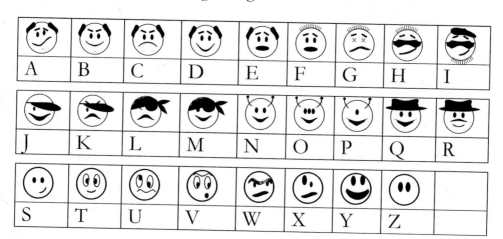

THE FUTURE

WILL BE

BETTER

TOMORROW

-- Dan Quayle

Time: min. _____ sec. _____

179

XI. Name as many state capitals as you can in one minute.

_____   _____

_____   _____

_____   _____

_____   _____

_____   _____

_____   _____

_____   _____

_____   _____

XII. Write as many of the To-Do list items as you can remember.

_____

_____

_____

_____

_____

_____

_____

XIII. Write as much as you can of the Fact of the Day.

_____

_____

_____

_____

I. Word Matrix (Find the following words in the matrix.)

1. COLORADO
2. IDAHO
3. KENTUCKY
4. MARYLAND
5. NEW YORK
6. TENNESEE
7. WISCONSIN
8. MISSOURI
9. MISSISSIPPI
10. CALIFORNIA

```
W H J I R U O S S I M C
A I N R O F I L A C M O
W L I H U V G D Y I Y L
I I W L R P Q K S K L O
S D X K Y Y C S M R Z R
C A Z C Y U I A D O D A
O H K T T S R D H Y H D
N O H N S Y P F M W A O
S E E I L P R U C E U T
I K P A S E R K Y N I E
N P N A E E S E N N E T
I D D W S I K Q M N M G
```

Time: min.____ sec. ____

II. Shopping List(Read aloud, cover, repeat aloud -- three times.)

salmon
asparagus
artichokes
grapefruit
pancake mix
lemons
potatoes
apricots
vegetable soup
tomatoes

III. Fact of the Day (Read aloud, cover, and say aloud -- three times.)

The National Park Service of the United States, which was created on August 25, 1916, oversees 58 national parks and many other areas such as national monuments, historical parks, national memorials, national recreation areas, and wild and scenic rivers.

IV. Write as many of the Shopping List items as you can remember.

_____   _____

_____   _____

_____   _____

_____   _____

_____   _____

V. Write as much as you can of the Fact of the Day.

_____

_____

_____

_____

VI. Word Chains

shun   bait

_____   _____

_____   _____

_____   _____

_____   _____

slug   _____

                mice

Time: min.____ sec. ____

VII. Coding: Decode the message using the code table.

A	B	C	D	E	F	G	H	I	J

K	L	M	N	O	P	Q	R	S	T

U	V	W	X	Y	Z	,	.	'	?

_ _ _ _ _ _ _ _ _ _ _ _ _ _

_ _ _ _ _ _ _ _

_ _ _ _ _ _ _ _ _ _ _ _

_ _ _ _ _ _ _ _ _ _ _

-- Richard Pryor

Time: min. _____ sec._____

VIII. Schedule

orig	dest	depart	arrive	flt#
DTW	SFO	9:22a	11:25a	343
DTW	SFO	12:15p	2:22p	345
DTW	SFO	7:39p	9:51p	347
FRA	DTW	10:20a	1:55p	51
SFO	NRT	12:00p	4:30p*	27

city	code	time
Detroit	DTW	GMT-5
Frankfurt	FRA	GMT+1
San Francisco	SFO	GMT-8
Tokyo	NRT	GMT+9
* next day		

a) How long is the flight from Frankfurt to Detroit?_____

b) Continuing on to Tokyo, what is the time in Frankfurt when you arrive in

   Tokyo?_____

Time: min. _____sec._____

IX. Complete the following sequences.

94	92	88	80	64	_____
C	D	F	I	M	_____
ZA	BY	XC	DW	VE	_____
D	C	E	B	F	_____
92129	83138	74147	65156	56165	_____

Time: min. _____sec._____

Brain Agility Exercises

X. Count the number of each symbol.

Time: min. _____ sec. _____

XI. Name as many items in the news as you can in one minute.

_____	_____
_____	_____
_____	_____
_____	_____
_____	_____
_____	_____
_____	_____
_____	_____
_____	_____
_____	_____

XII. Write as many of the Shopping List items as you can remember.

_____	_____
_____	_____
_____	_____
_____	_____
_____	_____

XIII. Write as much as you can of the Fact of the Day.

_____

_____

_____

_____

Brain Agility Exercises

I. Complete the following sequences.

99	96	91	84	75	_____
4	D	8	H	16	_____
97/16	91/10	85/13	79/16	73/10	_____
Z	26	W	23	T	_____
B	C	E	H	L	_____

Time: min. _____ sec. _____

II. Shopping List(Read aloud, cover, repeat aloud -- three times.)

   watermelon
   baking soda
   pork roast
   garlic
   leeks
   eggs
   cottage cheese
   pancake mix
   grapefruit
   swiss chard

III. Fact of the Day (Read aloud, cover, and say aloud -- three times.)

The world's earliest known astronomical megalith accurately marking the summer solstice was built before 5000 BC at Nabata Playa, 500 miles south of modern day Cairo. It is 1000 years older than Stonehenge.

IV. Write as many of the Shopping List items as you can remember.

_____   _____

_____   _____

_____   _____

_____   _____

_____   _____

V. Write as much as you can of the Fact of the Day.

_____

_____

_____

_____

VI. Word Chains

hill   slick

_____   _____

_____   _____

_____   _____

_____   _____

road   skate

Time: min.____ sec. ____

VII. Find the figures which are rotations and not reflections of the figure
　　　at the left of each line.

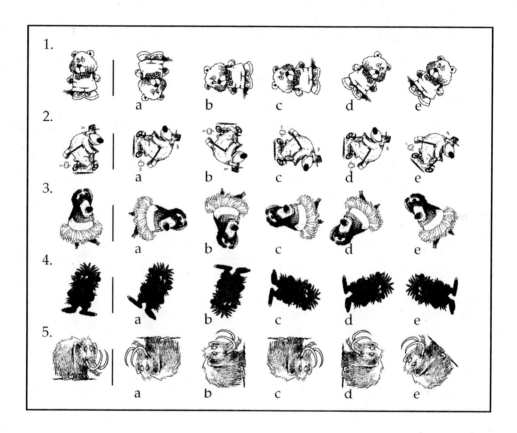

1)_____ 2)_____ 3)_____ 4)_____ 5)_____

Time: min.____ sec. ____

VIII. Calculate the following:

42433	11411	34158	39774	65977
10466	22164	2999	42609	85302

98393	83611	80064	81409	75940
-17602	-65948	-19290	-77282	-56336

Time: min.____ sec. ____

IX. Find as many words of three letters or more which can be made from the letters of the following word. (Time limit - 3 minutes)

AUSTRALIA

_____	_____
_____	_____
_____	_____
_____	_____
_____	_____
_____	_____
_____	_____

X. Count the number of each symbol.

∩___ ↺___ ↰___ ↻___

Time: min. _____sec._____

XI. Name as many politicians as you can in one minute.

_____   _____

_____   _____

_____   _____

_____   _____

_____   _____

_____   _____

_____   _____

_____   _____

_____   _____

_____   _____

XII. Write as many of the Shopping List items as you can remember.

_____   _____

_____   _____

_____   _____

_____   _____

_____   _____

XIII. Write as much as you can of the Fact of the Day.

_____

_____

_____

_____

I. Word Matrix (Find the following words in the matrix.)

1. CEREBELLUM
2. CORTEX
3. FRONTAL
4. GLIAL
5. NEURON
6. OCCIPITAL
7. SYNAPSE
8. TEMPORAL
9. THALAMUS
10. HIPPOCAMPUS

```
S U P M A C O P P I H N
T T M L V F U K F H Q E
L X H U U Y N K T Y A C
A G E S L D N O R U E N
R L A T Y L Q V V Y C P
O I J K R N E L V N X X
P A P S I O A B Q F A L
M L T Y G T C P E C M Z
E O P N N G O Z S R A Y
T A S O W O P H E E E T
B Q R T H A L A M U S C
W F X O C C I P I T A L
```

Time: min.____ sec. ____

II. To-Do List(Read aloud, cover, repeat aloud -- three times.)

phone insurance agent
buy batteries for camera
plant flowers
get bus schedule
special on TV tonight
go to talk on health insurance
renew prescription

III. Fact of the Day (Read aloud, cover, and say aloud -- three times.)

The four longest rivers in the world are: Nile (4,181 mi.), Amazon (4,032 mi.), Mississippi-Missouri (3,919 mi.), and Yangtze (3,903 mi.).

IV. Write as many of the To-Do list items as you can remember.

_____

_____

_____

_____

_____

_____

_____

V. Write as much as you can of the Fact of the Day.

_____

_____

_____

_____

VI. Schedule

orig	dest	depart	arrive	flt#	city	code	time
BKK	NRT	6:00a	1:50p	28	Bangkok	BKK	GMT+7
NRT	SEA	3:25p	7:15a	8	Minneapolis	MSP	GMT-6
SEA	MSP	7:00a	12:16p	806	Seattle	SEA	GMT-8
SEA	MSP	8:55a	2:07p	158	Tokyo	NRT	GMT+9
SEA	MSP	12:20p	5:33p	170			
SEA	MSP	3:11p	9:23p	164			

Note that due to the time differences the arrival time may be earlier than the departure time -- on the same day. This happens when crossing the date line.

a) What is the shortest travel time from Bangkok to Minneapolis?_____

b) How long is the flight from Bangkok to Tokyo?_____

                                    Time: min. _____sec._____

Brain Agility Exercises

VII. Find the figures which are rotations and not reflections of the figure at the left of each line.

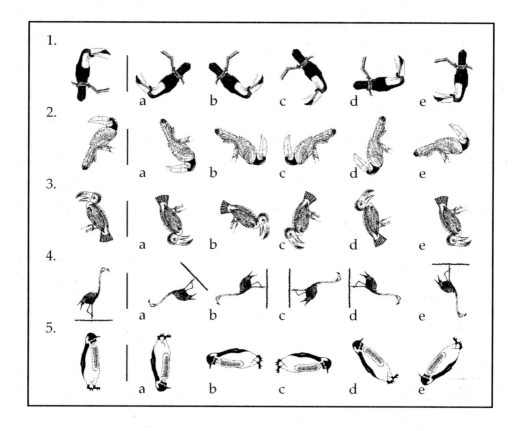

1)_____ 2)_____ 3)_____ 4)_____ 5)_____

Time: min. _____sec._____

VIII. Calculate the following:

92060	10719	43337	42103	14859
31485	43110	30073	95788	40809

72185	76103	48571	63866	82941
-54206	-35438	-38560	-46996	-45592

Time: min. _____sec._____

IX. Find as many words of three letters or more which can be made from the letters of the following word. (Time limit - 3 minutes)

AEROBICS

_____   _____

_____   _____

_____   _____

_____   _____

_____   _____

_____   _____

_____   _____

Brain Agility Exercises

X. Coding: Decode the message using the code table.

⇨	⇦	⇨	⇦	⇨	←	→	↑	↓	↖
A	B	C	D	E	F	G	H	I	J

↗	↙	↘	↔	↕	▲	▼	△	▽	◀
K	L	M	N	O	P	Q	R	S	T

▶	◁	▷	◣	◤	◢	⊥	↘	⇦	⌐
U	V	W	X	Y	Z	,	.	'	?

⇨   ← ⇨ ↔ ⇨ ◀ ↓ ⇨   ↓ ▽

A — _ _ _ _ _ _ _ — _ _

↕ ↔ ⇨   ▷ ↑ ↕   ⇨ ⇨ ↔ ⇦ ◀

_ _ _ — _ _ _ — _ _ _ _ _

⇨ ↑ ⇨ ↔ → ⇨   ↑ ↓ ▽   ↘ ↓ ↔ ⇦

_ _ _ _ _ _ — _ _ _ — _ _ _ _

⇨ ↔ ⇦   ▷ ↕ ↔ ⇦ ◀   ⇨ ↑ ⇨ ↔ → ⇨

_ _ _ — _ _ _ _ _ — _ _ _ _ _ _

◀ ↑ ⇨   ▽ ▶ ⇦ ↖ ⇨ ⇨ ◀ ↘

_ _ _ — _ _ _ _ _ _ _ _

-- Winston Churchill

Time: min.____ sec. ____

197

XI. Name as many weather conditions as you can in one minute.

_____   _____
_____   _____
_____   _____
_____   _____
_____   _____
_____   _____
_____   _____

XII. Write as many of the To-Do list items as you can remember.

_____
_____
_____
_____
_____
_____
_____

XIII. Write as much as you can of the Fact of the Day.

_____
_____
_____
_____

Brain Agility Exercises

I. Word Matrix (Find the following words in the matrix.)

1. ANKARA
2. BAGHDAD
3. BANGKOK
4. BUDAPEST
5. BUENOS AIRES
6. DUBLIN
7. REYKJAVIK
8. SANTIAGO
9. WARSAW
10. PRAGUE

```
V H E V S S C N Q P R P
S K B A G H D A D E W F
E I T G S Y I U O A L S
R V G Q I P B Q S C A P
I A L D B L R R M N Q B
A J T A I U A A T G A J
S K B N C W D I G N B X
O Y O K N I A A G U V K
N E K A O G W K P F E M
E R B R O G O F H E Q N
U F J A G K O T T F S C
B L C E A J O I A N F T
```

Time: min.____ sec. ____

II. Shopping List(Read aloud, cover, repeat aloud -- three times.)

flour
clam chowder
peaches
cherries
milk
squash
jam
vegetable soup
napkins
tea

III. Fact of the Day (Read aloud, cover, and say aloud -- three times.)

There are currently 205 planets known to exist in solar systems outside of our solar system. The largest of these extra-solar planetary systems has four planets discovered in August 2004.

IV. Write as many of the Shopping List items as you can remember.

_____   _____

_____   _____

_____   _____

_____   _____

_____   _____

V. Write as much as you can of the Fact of the Day.

_____

_____

_____

_____

VI. Word Chains

hand   salt

_____   _____

_____   _____

_____   _____

_____   _____

foot   food

Time: min.____ sec. ____

VII. Coding: Decode the message using the code table.

A	B	C	D	E	F	G	H	I

J	K	L	M	N	O	P	Q	R

S	T	U	V	W	X	Y	Z	

— — — — — — — —

— — — — — — — —

— — — — — — — — — — —

— — — — — — — — — — —

— — — — — — — — — —

— —

--Albert Einstein

Time: min. _____ sec. _____

VIII. Schedule

orig	dest	depart	arrive	flt#
DTW	SFO	9:22a	11:25a	343
DTW	SFO	12:15p	2:22p	345
DTW	SFO	7:39p	9:51p	347
JFK	DTW	9:02a	11:13a	898
JFK	DTW	12:35p	2:53p	894
JFK	DTW	4:11p	6:25p	896
NRT	PEK	5:55p	9:10p	11
SFO	NRT	12:00p	4:30p*	27

city	code	time
Beijing	PEK	GMT+7
Detroit	DTW	GMT-5
New York	JFK	GMT-5
San Francisco	SFO	GMT-8
Tokyo	NRT	GMT+9

* next day

a) Assuming you will stay overnight in San Francisco, what is the latest you can leave New York to travel to Beijing?_____

b) How long is the flight from Tokyo to Beijing?_____

c) What is the total travel time from San Francisco to Beijing?_____

Time: min. _____sec._____

IX. Complete the following sequences.

2   5   10   17   26   _____

AB   BD   CG   DK   EP   _____

5   6   9   10   13   _____

BA   ED   HG   KJ   NM   _____

W   T   Q   N   K   _____

Time: min. _____sec._____

X. Count the number of each symbol.

Time: min. _____ sec. _____

XI. Name as many uses of paper as you can in one minute.

_____   _____

_____   _____

_____   _____

_____   _____

_____   _____

_____   _____

_____   _____

_____   _____

_____   _____

XII. Write as many of the Shopping List items as you can remember.

_____   _____

_____   _____

_____   _____

_____   _____

_____   _____

XIII. Write as much as you can of the Fact of the Day.

_____

_____

_____

_____

I. Complete the following sequences.

19	82	37	64	55	_____
YB	ZA	WD	XC	UF	_____
1023	1019	1009	999	981	_____
A	C	F	J	O	_____
Y	V	S	P	M	_____

Time: min. _____ sec. _____

II. Shopping List(Read aloud, cover, repeat aloud -- three times.)

bath soap
cauliflower
potatoes
broccoli
bread
grape jam
squash
ham
milk
zucchini

III. Fact of the Day (Read aloud, cover, and say aloud -- three times.)

The first Nobel Peace Prize was awarded in 1901 to Jean Henri
Dunant (Switzerland) founder of the Red Cross and initiator of the
Geneva Convention. Other recipients have been H.H. Dalai Lama,
1989, and Bishop Desmond Tutu, 1984.

IV. Write as many of the Shopping List items as you can remember.

_____   _____

_____   _____

_____   _____

_____   _____

_____   _____

V. Write as much as you can of the Fact of the Day.

_____

_____

_____

_____

VI. Word Chains

past   lose

_____   _____

_____   _____

_____   _____

_____   _____

_____   _____

time   find

Time: min.____ sec. ____

VII. Find the figures which are rotations and not reflections of the figure
     at the left of each line.

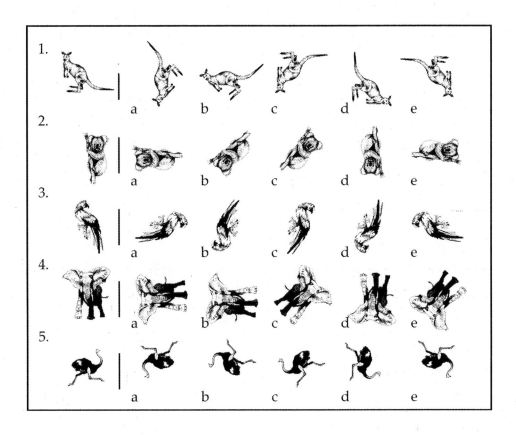

1)_____ 2)_____ 3)_____ 4)_____ 5)_____

Time: min.____ sec. ____

VIII. Calculate the following:

84286	71443	15653	87291	78365
77617	14133	89630	18538	67619

46648	62749	61112	92120	75540
-32140	-45701	-45916	-86592	-62932

Time: min.____ sec. ____

IX. Find as many words of three letters or more which can be made from the letters of the following word. (Time limit - 3 minutes)

TELEVISION

_____   _____

_____   _____

_____   _____

_____   _____

_____   _____

_____   _____

_____   _____

Brain Agility Exercises

X. Count the number of each symbol.

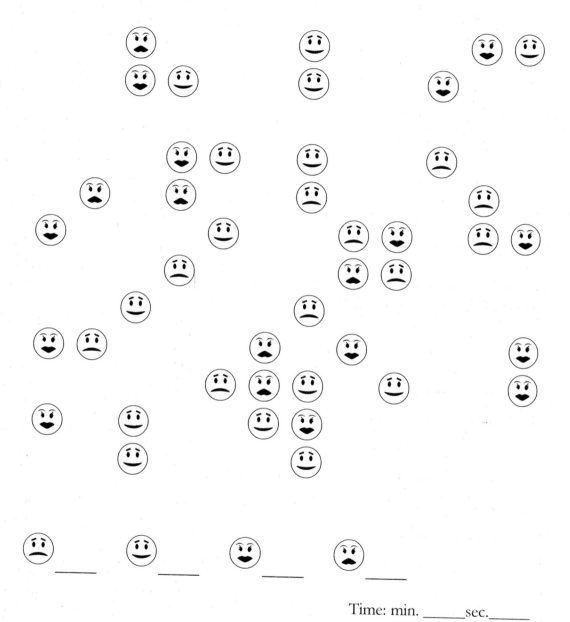

Time: min. _____sec._____

XI. Name as many authors as you can in one minute.

_____   _____

_____   _____

_____   _____

_____   _____

_____   _____

_____   _____

_____   _____

_____   _____

_____   _____

_____   _____

XII. Write as many of the Shopping List items as you can remember.

_____   _____

_____   _____

_____   _____

_____   _____

_____   _____

XIII. Write as much as you can of the Fact of the Day.

_____

_____

_____

_____

I. Word Matrix (Find the following words in the matrix.)

1. CD ROM
2. FLOPPY
3. GLITCH
4. MEMORY
5. MODEM
6. HARD DRIVE
7. KEYBOARD
8. PRINTER
9. SOFTWARE
10. MONITOR

```
E V I R D D R A H N A H
K O P Y X I E E H C C S
C E M F I B R B X T C V
E X Y M A A V E I M P I
A L O B W G M L Y F A B
F R K T O O G M S M F X
R L F D D A J D O X W B
W O O E V L R N W R V J
S P M P S H I D C M D L
R A O Q P T A C O P B C
P O M J O Y R O M E M U
J D P R R E T N I R P U
```

Time: min.____ sec. ____

II. To-Do List(Read aloud, cover, repeat aloud -- three times.)

buy batteries for camera
recycle newspapers
wrap and mail package
water garden
cancel airline tickets
recycle bottles
have eyeglass frames adjusted

III. Fact of the Day (Read aloud, cover, and say aloud -- three times.)

With a population just over 300 million, Americans constitute 5% of the world's population and consume 25% of the world's resources.

IV. Write as many of the To-Do list items as you can remember.

_____

_____

_____

_____

_____

_____

_____

V. Write as much as you can of the Fact of the Day.

_____

_____

_____

_____

VI. Schedule

orig	dest	depart	arrive	flt#	city	code	time
HKG	NRT	8:45a	1:30p	2	Hong Kong	HKG	GMT+8
NRT	SEA	3:25p	7:15a	8	Minneapolis	MSP	GMT-6
SEA	MSP	3:11p	9:23p	164	Seattle	SEA	GMT-8
					Tokyo	NRT	GMT+9

a) How long is the flight from Hong Kong to Tokyo?_____

b) How long is the flight from Tokyo to Seattle?_____

c) What is the time in Hong Kong when you arrive in Seattle?_____

Time: min. _____sec._____

VII. Find the figures which are rotations and not reflections of the figure at the left of each line.

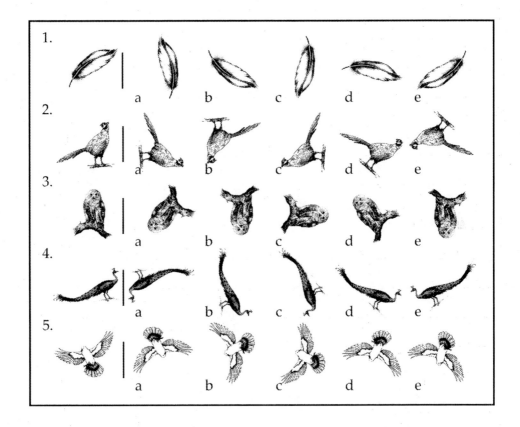

1)_____ 2)_____ 3)_____ 4)_____ 5)_____

Time: min. _____sec._____

VIII. Calculate the following:

12814	32459	60436	41613	21926
17990	45022	2798	76913	60156

78723	64016	63783	90677	82148
-12504	-35619	-35676	-67105	-56036

Time: min. _____sec._____

IX. Find as many words of three letters or more which can be made from the letters of the following word. (Time limit - 3 minutes)

CASTLE

_____	_____
_____	_____
_____	_____
_____	_____
_____	_____
_____	_____
_____	_____

X. Coding: Decode the message using the code table.

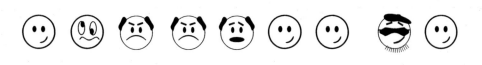

__ __ __ __ __ __ __ __ __

-- Woody Allen

Time: min.___ sec. ___

XI. Name as many forms of transportation as you can in one minute.

_____   _____

_____   _____

_____   _____

_____   _____

_____   _____

_____   _____

_____   _____

_____   _____

XII. Write as many of the To-Do list items as you can remember.

_____

_____

_____

_____

_____

_____

_____

XIII. Write as much as you can of the Fact of the Day.

_____

_____

_____

_____

I. Word Matrix (Find the following words in the matrix.)

1. COMMITTEE
2. CONGRESS
3. LEGISLATOR
4. MAJORITY
5. PARLIAMENT
6. REPUBLICAN
7. SECRETARY
8. SENATE
9. SENATOR
10. DEMOCRAT

```
U  N  L  E  G  I  S  L  A  T  O  R
A  C  B  Q  V  L  P  L  H  N  T  C
U  O  N  O  U  O  K  T  A  N  O  S
U  M  O  O  Z  X  A  C  E  N  U  E
F  M  J  V  V  R  I  M  G  M  Z  N
Y  I  A  R  C  L  A  R  A  S  W  A
Y  T  Q  O  B  I  E  J  I  V  P  T
E  T  M  U  L  S  O  T  Z  C  B  O
Z  E  P  R  S  R  L  N  A  M  R  R
D  E  A  I  I  Z  Z  V  L  N  C  R
R  P  Y  T  V  J  D  Q  B  U  E  F
O  P  Y  R  A  T  E  R  C  E  S  S
```

Time: min.____ sec. ____

II. Shopping List(Read aloud, cover, repeat aloud -- three times.)

lamb chops
apricots
olive oil
oatmeal
ice cream
black pepper
tomato soup
watermelon
bok choy
baking soda

III. Fact of the Day (Read aloud, cover, and say aloud -- three times.)

Groundhog Day stems from a 5th century belief of the European Celts that animals had supernatural powers on the day half-way between the Winter Solstice and the Spring Equinox. The Romans observed Hedgehog Day.

IV. Write as many of the Shopping List items as you can remember.

_____　　_____

_____　　_____

_____　　_____

_____　　_____

_____　　_____

V. Write as much as you can of the Fact of the Day.

_____

_____

_____

_____

VI. Word Chains

kiss　　　　　　slow

_____　　　　　_____

_____　　　　　_____

_____　　　　　_____

_____　　　　　_____

_____　　　　　_____

toad　　　　　　fast

Time: min.____ sec. ____

VII. Coding: Decode the message using the code table.

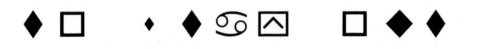

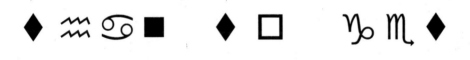

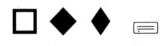

A	B	C	D	E	F	G	H	I
♋	♌	♍	♎	♏	♐	♑	♒	♓

J	K	L	M	N	O	P	Q	R
er	&	●	◐	■	□	□	□	□

S	T	U	V	W	X	Y	Z	.
◆	◆	◆	❖	◆	⊠	⟁	⌘	▭

Decoded message:

IT IS EASIER

TO STAY OUT

THAN TO GET

OUT.

-- Mark Twain

Time: min. _____ sec. _____

VIII. Schedule

orig	dest	depart	arrive	flt#
DTW	SFO	9:22a	11:25a	343
DTW	SFO	12:15p	2:22p	345
DTW	SFO	7:39p	9:51p	347
NRT	HKG	6:20p	10:35p	1
SFO	NRT	12:00p	4:30p*	27

city	code	time
Detroit	DTW	GMT-5
Hong Kong	HKG	GMT+8
San Francisco	SFO	GMT-8
Tokyo	NRT	GMT+9

* next day

a) Assuming you need only 30 min. transit time in San Francisco, what is the latest you can leave Detroit for Hong Kong?_____

b) What is the total travel time from Detroit to Hong Kong?_____

c) How long is the flight from Tokyo to Hong Kong?_____

Time: min. _____sec._____

IX. Complete the following sequences.

927　836　745　654　563　_____

CB　AD　EZ　YF　GX　_____

11　24　39　56　75　_____

AB　BD　CF　DH　EJ　_____

YA　VC　SE　PG　MI　_____

Time: min. _____sec._____

X. Count the number of each symbol.

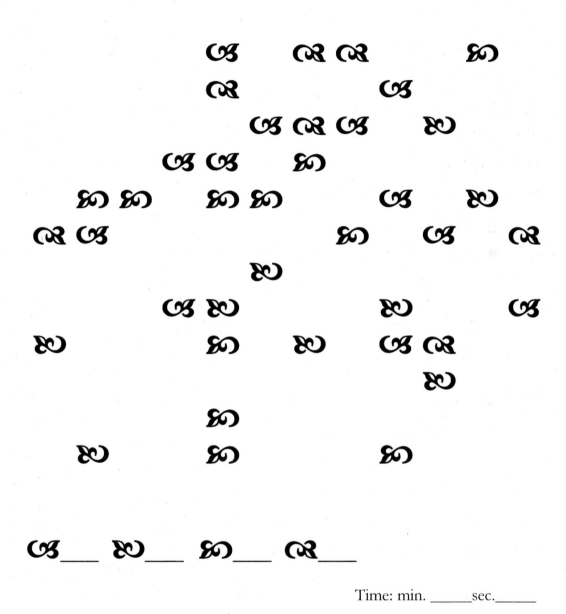

XI. Name as many artists as you can in one minute.

    _____   _____

    _____   _____

    _____   _____

    _____   _____

    _____   _____

    _____   _____

    _____   _____

    _____   _____

    _____   _____

XII. Write as many of the Shopping List items as you can remember.

    _____   _____

    _____   _____

    _____   _____

    _____   _____

    _____   _____

XIII. Write as much as you can of the Fact of the Day.

_____

_____

_____

_____

Brain Agility Exercises

I. Complete the following sequences.

972 883 774 685 576 _____

MO PL KQ RJ IS _____

ABC CBD DBE EBF FBG _____

ABB CCD EFF GGH IJJ _____

WA VB TC QD ME _____

Time: min. _____ sec. _____

II. Shopping List(Read aloud, cover, repeat aloud -- three times.)

grapefruit
eggplant
soup
ham
applesauce
toothpaste
sirloin steak
spaghetti
green beans
cantaloupe

III. Fact of the Day (Read aloud, cover, and say aloud -- three times.)

Nepal, home to Mount Everest, the world's highest mountain, is a country of 28 million people situated between India and Tibet.

IV. Write as many of the Shopping List items as you can remember.

_____   _____

_____   _____

_____   _____

_____   _____

_____   _____

V. Write as much as you can of the Fact of the Day.

_____

_____

_____

_____

VI. Word Chains

take   book

_____   _____

_____   _____

_____   _____

_____   _____

_____   _____

fool   page

Time: min.____ sec. ____

VII. Find the figures which are rotations and not reflections of the figure
    at the left of each line.

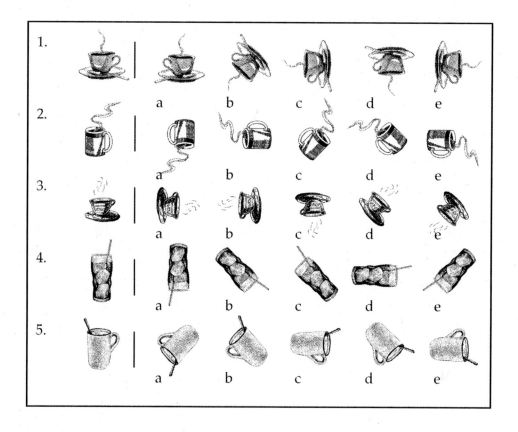

1)_____ 2)_____ 3)_____ 4)_____ 5)_____

Time: min.____ sec. ____

VIII. Calculate the following:

50860	83782	67426	39734	36250
24719	37120	67207	97627	21201

63045	77049	27744	72031	95031
-51970	-30083	-10240	-38284	-23867

Time: min.____ sec. ____

IX. Find as many words of three letters or more which can be made from the letters of the following word. (Time limit - 3 minutes)

INTELLIGENCE

_____	_____
_____	_____
_____	_____
_____	_____
_____	_____
_____	_____
_____	_____

X. Count the number of each symbol.

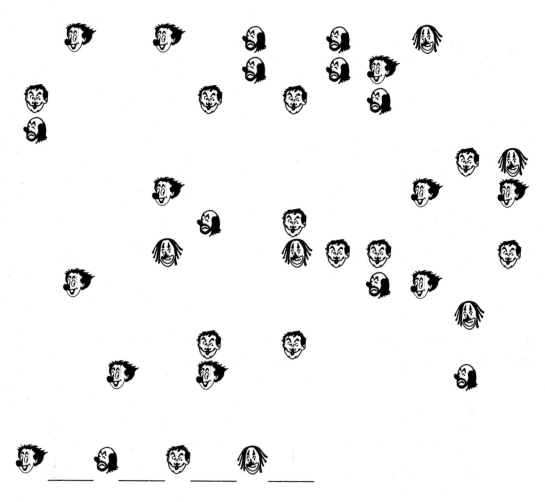

Time: min. _____ sec._____

XI. Name as many government offices as you can in one minute.

_____   _____

_____   _____

_____   _____

_____   _____

_____   _____

_____   _____

_____   _____

_____   _____

_____   _____

_____   _____

XII. Write as many of the Shopping List items as you can remember.

_____   _____

_____   _____

_____   _____

_____   _____

_____   _____

XIII. Write as much as you can of the Fact of the Day.

_____

_____

_____

_____

I. Word Matrix (Find the following words in the matrix.)

1. AMAZON
2. COLORADO
3. CONGO
4. DANUBE
5. GANGES
6. RHINE
7. SEINE
8. URAL
9. YANGTZE
10. ZAMBEZI

```
A I L C G A Z N D B J B
E I J G E B U N A D N Z
B Z G A N G E S X O C S
S E D A S A X Y Z O K M
C B D A E U Y A L S L Q
F M H W I A M O S M O S
B A F N N A R L M R M P
S Z S G E A R H I N E V
C V T U D Q M O Q Q Z F
O Z G O R B S A K L J Z
E M C Q Q A C O N G O O
W E C V J O L G K F E T
```

Time: min.____ sec. ____

II. To-Do List(Read aloud, cover, repeat aloud -- three times.)

register for evening class
call electrician
luncheon appointment
recycle newspapers
buy fish food
do brain agility exercises
put out trash

III. Fact of the Day (Read aloud, cover, and say aloud -- three times.)

In 2007 seven of the prognosticating groundhogs in the United States predicted an early spring while four groundhogs predicted six more weeks of winter.

IV. Write as many of the To-Do list items as you can remember.

_____

_____

_____

_____

_____

_____

_____

V. Write as much as you can of the Fact of the Day.

_____

_____

_____

_____

VI. Schedule

orig	dest	depart	arrive	flt#
MSP	MIA	7:15p	11:42p	568
NRT	SEA	3:25p	7:15a	8
PEK	NRT	9:05a	1:40p	12
SEA	MSP	8:55a	2:07p	158

city	code	time
Beijing	PEK	GMT+7
Miami	MIA	GMT-5
Minneapolis	MSP	GMT-6
Seattle	SEA	GMT-8
Tokyo	NRT	GMT+9

a) What is the total travel time from Beijing to Miami?_____

b) What is the total time in the air from Beijing to Seattle?_____

c) What time is it in Beijing when you arrive in Miami?_____

Time: min. _____sec._____

VII. Find the figures which are rotations and not reflections of the figure at the left of each line.

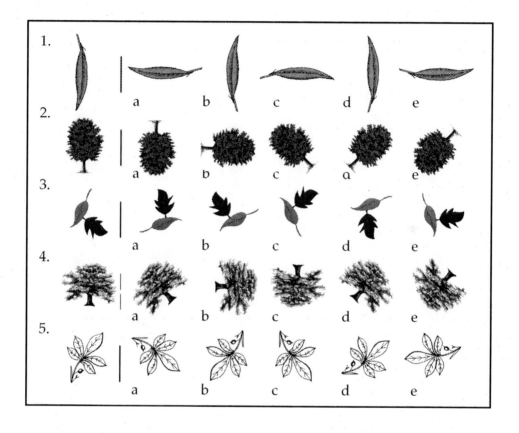

1)_____ 2)_____ 3)_____ 4)_____ 5)_____

Time: min. _____sec._____

VIII. Calculate the following:

291557	52966	67699	67471	14271
76178	56509	51387	89298	18618

68362	13304	33793	84347	87002
-22068	-12662	-26713	-32815	-71540

Time: min. _____sec._____

IX. Find as many words of three letters or more which can be made from the letters of the following word. (Time limit - 3 minutes)

RECREATION

_____	_____
_____	_____
_____	_____
_____	_____
_____	_____
_____	_____
_____	_____

X. Coding: Decode the message using the code table.

⇨	⇦	⇨	⇦	⇨	←	→	↑	↓	↖
A	B	C	D	E	F	G	H	I	J

↗	↙	↘	↔	↕	▲	▼	△	▽	◀
K	L	M	N	O	P	Q	R	S	T

▶	◁	▷	◣	◤	▼	↓	↘	⇦	↴
U	V	W	X	Y	Z	,	.	'	?

◀ ⇨ ↙ ⇨ ◁ ↓ ▽ ↓ ↕ ↔   ↓ ▽

_ _ _ _ _ _ _ _ _ _   _ _

◀ ↑ ⇨   ◀ △ ↓ ▶ ↘ ▲ ↑

_ _ _   _ _ _ _ _ _ _

↕ ←   ↘ ⇨ ⇨ ↑ ↓ ↔ ⇨

_ _   _ _ _ _ _ _ _

↕ ◁ ⇨ △   ▲ ⇨ ↕ ▲ ↙ ⇨ ↘

_ _ _ _   _ _ _ _ _ _ _

-- Fred Allen

Time: min.____ sec. ____

XI. Name as many books as you can in one minute.

_____   _____

_____   _____

_____   _____

_____   _____

_____   _____

_____   _____

_____   _____

_____   _____

XII. Write as many of the To-Do list items as you can remember.

_____

_____

_____

_____

_____

_____

_____

XIII. Write as much as you can of the Fact of the Day.

_____

_____

_____

_____

I. Word Matrix (Find the following words in the matrix.)

1. CARPENTER
2. DOCTOR
3. ENGINEER
4. JANITOR
5. JUDGE
6. PILOT
7. POLICE
8. SOLDIER
9. TINKER
10. TEACHER

```
A B D X R M Q K S Q T L
R E H C A E T A R V I R
O D O C T O R E E V N E
P Z R R T O Z G T M K E
E S W Z O J J D N M E N
T J M H P T B U E M R I
V K W I S P I J P B B G
G N L P S O J N R P R N
P O S Y Z L B O A P A E
T S O L D I E R C J E Q
A C N X Y C O U N P F S
H D E G K E T B Y Y O C
```

Time: min.____ sec. ____

II. Shopping List(Read aloud, cover, repeat aloud -- three times.)

chicken
olive oil
paper toweling
squash
pickles
flour
potatoes
mustard
cranberry sauce
peanut butter

III. Fact of the Day (Read aloud, cover, and say aloud -- three times.)

Researchers at the University of Indiana found that four 10-minute
walks spread out over a day reduced blood pressure for 10 to 11
hours -- about three hours longer than a single nonstop 40 minute walk.

IV. Write as many of the Shopping List items as you can remember.

_____   _____

_____   _____

_____   _____

_____   _____

_____   _____

V. Write as much as you can of the Fact of the Day.

_____

_____

_____

_____

VI. Word Chains

stone   lamp

_____   _____

_____   _____

_____   _____

_____   _____

_____   _____

_____   _____

clams   _____

               _____

               bulb

Time: min.____ sec. ____

VII. Coding: Decode the message using the code table.

A	B	C	D	E	F	G	H	I	J

K	L	M	N	O	P	Q	R	S	T

U	V	W	X	Y	Z	,	.	'	?

— — — — — — — — — — —

— — — — — — — — —

— — — — — — — —

— — — — — — — — — —

-- Confucius

Time: min. _____sec._____

237

VIII. Schedule

orig	dest	depart	arrive	flt#	city	code	time
DTW	FRA	5:00p	7:20a*	52	Detroit	DTW	GMT-5
HNL	SEA	2:10p	9:45p	220	Frankfurt	FRA	GMT+1
HNL	SEA	10:00p	5:35a*	806	Honolulu	HNL	GMT-10
SEA	DTW	8:40a	3:54p	210	Seattle	SEA	GMT-8
SEA	DTW	12:30p	7:40p	250			
SEA	DTW	10:06p	5:06a*	208	*next day		

a) How long is the flight from Detroit to Frankfurt?_____

b) How long is flight 806?_____

c) What time is it in Honolulu when you arrive in Frankfurt?_____

Time: min. _____sec._____

IX. Complete the following sequences.

11	23	34	46	57	_____
ACEG	BDFH	CEGI	DFHJ	EGIK	_____
WY	SU	OQ	KM	GI	_____
AEB	BFC	CGD	DHE	EIF	_____
1	3	6	10	15	_____

Time: min. _____sec._____

X. Count the number of each symbol.

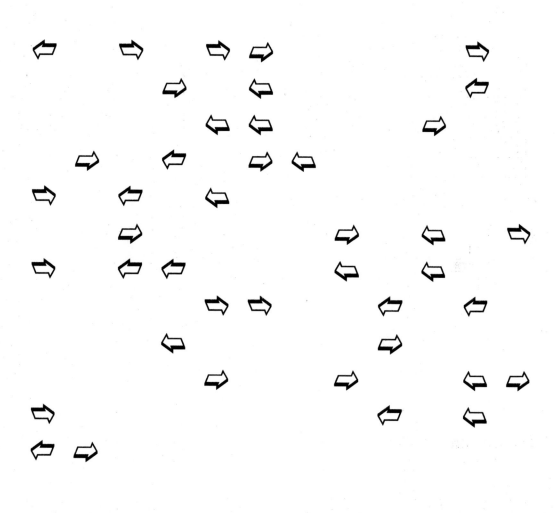

XI. Name as many holidays as you can in one minute.

_____	_____
_____	_____
_____	_____
_____	_____
_____	_____
_____	_____
_____	_____
_____	_____
_____	_____
_____	_____

XII. Write as many of the Shopping List items as you can remember.

_____	_____
_____	_____
_____	_____
_____	_____
_____	_____

XIII. Write as much as you can of the Fact of the Day.

_____

_____

_____

_____

CONGRATULATIONS, YOU HAVE FINISHED THE EXERCISES!

Continuing Mental Exercise   11

When you have completed the 30 day program of Brain Agility exercises and experience the benefits of mental exercise, you will likely wonder, "Where do I go from here?" Keeping mentally active is essential for brain health. Continuing some form of mental exercise can be an important part of this activity. There are many possibilities which are discussed below and included in the section Further Reading and Resources.

Paper and Pencil Puzzles are found in most local newspapers and are available in inexpensive puzzle books. Currently, the most popular seem to be crossword puzzles, Sudoku, and word puzzles such as Jumble and Cryptoquote. Puzzle books of numeric puzzles, logic puzzles, and word puzzles abound in newsstands and bookstores.

Please keep in mind that variety is very important. While being addicted to one type of puzzle is still of benefit, cognitive functions not challenged by that particular puzzle may be neglected.

Card games can also provide good cognitive challenges. Joining a bridge group will offer social interaction as well as excellent mental activity. If you want to work by yourself, solitaire comes in many forms. Free Cell is a version of solitaire that is being used to predict the onset of dementia by researchers at Oregon Health Sciences University in collaboration with Spry Learning in Portland, Oregon.(57) Free Cell is part of the game packages provided with Windows™ and other computer operating systems. Another card game that can be played by one or more is SET™. This is a quite different card game that exercises concept formation and processing speed. It is also available as a computer game, both for stand alone computers and on the internet.(58)

Electronic games provide interaction that can be challenging and entertaining. Some are dedicated to particular puzzles such as Sudoku or Minesweeper. Others provide suites of several games. The hand-held electronic games cost in the range of $10 to $50. At the high end Nintendo offers two mental exercise programs, Brain Age™ and Big Brain™ for its DS Lite, pocket game device with a color display screen and a variety of input and output modalities. The cost is about $125 for the game device and $20 for each program.

Many, many computer games are available for mental exercise. These range from single games to suites of exercises addressing different cognitive functions. Many games such as the classic Minesweeper are packed as part of popular operating systems. While many computer games have a modest cost, many are freeware that can be downloaded from the internet free of cost.

Many web sites offer a variety of on-line internet games designed specifically for improving cognitive functioning. Some web sites offer suites of games of varying levels of difficulty. Some suites are available for internet use for a monthly subscription fee ranging from $5 to $10 per month. Other suites are sold on CDs or via downloading from the internet for a one-time cost ranging from $20 to $50.(59,60,61,62,63)

If you do find internet games interesting and challenging, it is important to monitor your use of them. There is growing concern about internet addiction and addiction to games. Some people become addicted to paper and pencil games such as Sudoku or solitaire card games. The interactive nature of the computer can make the attraction to computerized games even stronger. Some observers have suggested that addiction to the internet develops as a way of maintaining a higher level of brain arousal.

High end computer programs have been developed specifically for improving brain function.(64,65) These cost from $125 to $400. If you are thinking of purchasing one of these high end packages, you might consider the following:
- Price
- Limits on use – can the package be used by more than one person, can it be used only once or as many times as needed?
- Number of different exercises, what cognitive functions are exercised, what input and output modalities are used?
- Performance tracking -- is a record of times and scores kept for measuring progress?
- Program of exercises -- does the package provide a set of exercises for a given session or does the user select which exercises will be used?
- Adjustment of difficulty -- are there varying levels of difficulty and does the computer adjust difficulty according to the user's performance?
- Internet connection -- is this required in order to use the program?

Further Reading & Resources 12

Books

Brain Facts: a Primer on the Brain and Nervous System
Society for Neuroscience 2006, Washington, D.C.

The Aging Brain (Maps of the Mind), Lawrence J. Whalley
Columbia University Press 2003

Images of Mind, Michael I. Posner and Marcus E. Raichle
Scientific American Library, New York 1997

Yoga for Wimps, Miriam Austin
Sterling Books Publishing, Inc., New York 2000

The Memory Bible, Gary Small, M.D.
Hyperion, New York 2002

The Memory Prescription, Gary Small, M.D. with Gigi Vorgan
Hyperion, New York 2004

Stop Memory Loss, William Cone, Ph.D.
Matteson Books, Pacific Palisades, CA 2005

Organizations

AARP, 601 E Street N.W., Washington, DC. 20049
tel: 800.424.3410
<http://www.aarp.org>

Alzheimer's Association, 225 N. Michigan Ave., Floor 17, Chicago, IL 60601
tel: 800.272.3900
<http://www.alz.org>

American Society on Aging, 833 Market St., Suite 511, San Francisco, CA 94103
tel: 415.974.9600
<http://www.asaging.org>

National Institute on Aging, 31 Center Drive, MSC 2292, Building 31, Room 5C27, Bethesda MD 20892
tel: 800.222.2225
<http://www.nih.gov/nia>

Oasis Institute, 7710 Carondelet Ave., St. Louis, MO 63105
tel:314.862.2933
<http://www.oasisnet.org>

UCLA Center on Aging, 10945 Le Conte Ave., Suite 3119, Los Angeles CA 90095
tel:310.794.0676
<http://www.aging.ucla.edu>

References   13

1) Developmental influences on adult intelligence: the Seattle longitudinal study. K. Warner Schaie, Oxford University Press, New York, 2005

2) Park DC, et.al., Cerebral aging: integration of brain and behavioral models of cognitive function. Dialogues in Clinical Neuroscience 2001;3(3):151-165.

3) Ball KK, et.al., Aging and the brain. in *Principles and Practice of Behavioral Neurology and Neuropsychology*, W.B.Saunders Co. Philadelphia, PA

4) Rosenweig MR, Bennett EL, Psychobiology of plasticity: Effects of training and experience on brain and behavior. Behavioral Brain Research 1996;78:57-65.

5) Gage FH, Structural plasticity of the adult brain. Dialogues in Clinical Neuroscience 2002;6(2):135-141.

6) Schaie KW, Willis SL, Can Decline in Adult Intellectual Functioning be Reversed?. Dev Psych 1986;22(2):223-232.

7) Guenther VK, et.al., Long term improvements in cognitive performance through computer-assisted cognitive training: a pilot study in a residential home for older people. Aging & Mental Health 2003;7(3):200-206.

8) Mahncke HW, et.al., Memory enhancement in healthy older adults using a brain plasticity-based training program: A randomized controlled study. Proceedings of the National Academy of Sciences 2006 Aug;103(33):12523-12528.

9) Posner MI, Raichle ME, *Images of Mind*, Scientific American Library, New York 1997

10) Diamond MC, Successful aging of the healthy brain, presented at the First Joint Conference of the American Society on Aging and the National Council on the Aging, March 10, 2001, New Orleans, LA.

11) Diamond MC, et.al., On the brain of a scientist: Albert Einstein. Experimental Neurology 1985 Apr;88(1):198-204

12) Pereira AC, et.al., An *in vivo* correlate of exercise-induced neurogenesis in the adult dentate gyrus. Proceedings of the National Academy of Sciences 2007 Mar;104(13):5638-5643.

13) Salthouse TA, The processing-speed theory of adult age differences in cognition. Psychological Review 1996;103(3):403-428.

14) Edwards JD, et.al., The impact of speed of processing training on cognitive and everyday performance. Aging & Mental Health 2005 May;9(3):262-271.

15) Schaie KW, Willis SL, Cognitive training in the normal elderly. in *Plasticite Cereberal et Stimulation Cognitive*, Forettey and Boller F(eds.) Paris,1994

16) Willis SL, Schaie KW, Training the elderly on the ability factors of spatial orientation and inductive reasoning. Psychology and Aging 1986;1(3)239-247.

17) Ball KB, et.al., Effects of cognitive training interventions with older adults. Journal of the American Medical Association 2002;288:2271-2281.

18) Willis SL, et.al., Long-term effects of cognitive training on everyday functional outcomes in older adults. Journal of the American Medical Association 2006;296(23)2805-2814.

19) Kramer AF,et.al., Exercise, cognition and the aging brain. Journal of Applied Physiology 2006:101:1237-1242.

20) Posner MI, et.al., Brain mechanisms and learning of high level skills. presented at meeting on Brain and Education, Vatican City, November 2003.

21) Rogers WA, Fisk AD, Understanding the role of attention in cognitive aging research. in *Handbook of the Psychology of Aging*, Academic Press 2001

22) Hallgren N, et.al., Cognitive effects in dichotic speech testing in elderly persons. Ear and Hearing 2001 Apr;22(2):120-129.

23) Richardson ED, Marottoli RA, Visual attention and driving behaviors among community-living older persons. The Journals of Gerontology Series A: Biological Sciences and Medical Sciences 2003;58:M832-M836.

24) Broman AT, et.al., Divided visual attention as a predictor of bumping while walking: The Salisbury Eye Evaluation. Investigative Ophthalmology & Visual Science 2004 Sept;45(9):2955-2960.

25) Mayo Clinic Staff (2006), Yoga: Minimize stress, maximize flexibility and even more, <http://www.mayoclinic.com/health/yoga/CM00004>

26) Mayo Clinic Staff (2005),Tai Chi: Stress reduction, balance, agility and more, <http://www.mayoclinic.com/health/tai-chi/SA00087>

27) Wolf SL, et.al., Reducing frailty and falls in older persons: an investigation of Tai Chi and computerized balance training. Journal of the American Geriatric Society 1996;44(5):489-97

28) Bassuk SS, et.al., Social disengagement and incident cognitive decline in community-dwelling elderly persons. Annals of Internal Medicine 1999 Aug;131(3):131-174.

29) Seeman TE, et.al., Social relationships, social support, and patterns of cognitive aging in healthy, high-functioning older adults: MacArthur studies of successful aging. Health Psychol.2001 Jul;20(4):243-255.

30) Reiter RJ, Oxidative processes and antioxidative defense mechanisms in the aging brain. The Federation of American Societies for Experimental Biology Journal 1995 May;9:526-533.

31) Beckman KB., Ames BN, The free radical theory of aging matures. Physiological Reviews 1998 Apr;78: 547-581.

32) Shigenaga MK, et.al. Oxidative Damage and Mitochondrial Decay in Aging. Proceedings of the National Academy of Sciences, (91):10771-10778

33) National Institutes of Health Office of Dietary Supplements: < http://ods.od.nih.gov/>

34) United States Department of Agriculture, Agriculture Research Service: <http://www.ars.usda.gov/Services/docs.htm?docid=8964>

35) Morris MC, et.al., Dietary intake of antioxidant nutrients and the risk of incident Alzheimer disease in a biracial community study. Journal of the American Medical Association 2002 Jun;287(24):3230-3237.

36) Morris MC, et.al., Dietary niacin and the risk of incident Alzheimer disease and of cognitive decline. Journal of Neurology, Neurosurgery, and Psychiatry 2004 Aug;75(8):10993-1099.

37) Engelhart MJ, et.al., Dietary intake of antioxidants and risk of Alzheimer disease. Journal of the American Medical Association 2002 Jun;287(24):3223-3229.

38) Durga J,et.al., Folate and the methylenetetrahydrofolate reductase 677C-->T mutation correlate with cognitive performance. Neurobiology of Aging 2006 Feb;27(2):334-45.

39) Ringman JM, et al., A potential role of the curry spice curcumin in Alzheimer's disease. Current Alzheimer Research 2005 Apr;2(2):131-136.

40) Linus Pauling Institute, Oregon State University,Curcumin. <http://lpi.oregonstate.edu/infocenter/phytochemicals/curcumin/>

41) Ames BN, Liu J, Delaying the mitochondrial decay of aging with acetylcarnitine. Annals of the New York Academy of Sciences 2004 Nov;1033:108-116.

42) Hutchins H, Symposium highlights -- Omega-3 fatty acids: Recommendations for therapeutics and prevention. Medscape General Medicine 2005;7(4).

43) Omega-3 fatty acids and health. National Institutes of Health <http://dietary-supplements.info.nih.gov/FactSheets/ Omega3FattyAcidsandHealth_pf.asp>

44) Morris MC, et.al., Dietary Fats and the Risk of Incident Alzheimer Disease. Archives of Neurology 2003;60:194-200.

45) Schaefer EJ, et.al., Plasma phosphatidycholine docosahexaenoic acid content and risk of dementia and Alzheimer disease. Archives of Neurology 2006 Nov;63(11)1545-1550.

46) Dietary Guidelines for Americans, United States Department of Health and Human Services and the United States Department of Agriculture 2005,

<http://www.health.gov/dietaryguidelines> or U.S. Government Printing Office (1-866-512-1800) Stock Number 001-000-04718-3.

47) Eating Well, AARP
<http://www.aarp.org/health/staying_healthy/eating>.

48) Kivipelto M, et.al., Risk score for the prediction of dementia risk in 20 years among middle aged people: a longitudinal population-based study. Lancet Neurology 2006 Sept;(9):735-741.

49) Colcombe SJ, et.al., Cardiovascular fitness, cortical plasticity, and aging. Proceedings of the National Academy of Science 2004 Mar;101(9):3316-3321.

50) Laurin D, et.al, Physical activity and risk of cognitive impairment and dementia in elderly persons. Archives of Neurology 2001 Mar;58(3):498-504.

51) Wang L, et.al., Performance-based physical function and future dementia in older people. Archives of Internal Medicine 2006 May;166(10);1115-1120.

52) Newcomer JW, et.al., Decreased memory performance in healthy humans induced by stress-level cortisol treatment. Archives of General Psychiatry 1999 Jun; 56(6):527-533

53) McEwen BS, Stress and the aging hippocampus. Frontiers in Neurodendocrinology 1999;20:49-70.

54) Podewils LJ, et.al., Relationship of self-perceptions of memory and worry to objective measures of memory and cognition in the general population. Psychosomatics 2003 Dec;44:461-470.

55) Nelson A(ed.) Improving Memory: Understanding age-related memory loss. Harvard Medical School 2006.

56) Daselaar SM, et.al., Effects of healthy aging on hippocampal and rhinal memory functions: An event-related fMRI study. Cerebral Cortex 2006;16(12):1771-1782.

57) Computer Card Game Detects Cognitive Changes. Oregon Health Sciences University Press Release (July 17, 2006)
<http://www.ohsu.edu/ohsuedu/newspub/releases/071706dementia.cfm>

58) Set Enterprises, Inc. <http://www.setgame.com>

59) Happy Neuron <http://www.happy-neuron.com>

60) BrainBuilder.com <http://www.brainbuilder.com>

61) Advanced Brain Technologies, LLC <http://www.advancedbrain.com>

62) Mindscape <http://www.mindscape.com.au>

63) Games for the Brain <http://www.gamesforthebrain.com>

64) PositScience <http://www.positscience.com

65) CogniFit <http://www.cognifit.com>

Solutions to Exercises 14

I. 11, 3, 24, 18, 5

VI. Note: there may be other solutions.

snare	**mall**	**pile**	**boar**
spare	*ball*	*pine*	*bear*
spore	*bale*	*nine*	*beat*
sport	**bane**	**none**	**meat**

VII. 1) a,c,e　2) a,c,d　3) a,c　4) a,b,e　5) a,b,d

VIII.

89493	51104	10286	119455	88883
92766	141812	69857	110912	88002

IX. BRAN, RAIN, AIR, BAN, BAR, BIN, NAB, NIB, RAN, RIB

X. + 9, - 11, o 13

I.

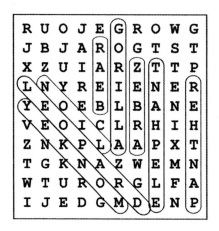

VI. a) 10:00am   b) 10:55am

VII. 1) a,c,d   2) a,d,e   3) a,b,e   4) b,c,d   5) a,b,e

VIII.   167404   111099   173041   171205   104956
           85616   51140   110197   147867   62897

IX. DENSE, NEEDS, SEWED, SWEDE, WEEDS, WEENS, WENDS, DENS, ENDS, EWES, NEED, NEWS, SEED, SEEN, SEND, SEWN, WEDS, WEED, WEEN, WEND

X. He who hesitates is sometimes saved.

I.

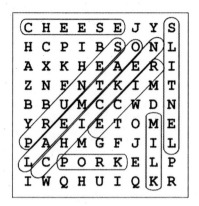

VI.

look	fill	stick	stars
took	*file*	*slick*	*stare*
tool	*fine*	*slice*	*spare*
fool	**wine**	**spice**	**spark**

VII. Age is a high price to pay for maturity.

VIII. a) 6:04am   b) 5:22pm or 17:22

IX. 30, 23, 27, 20, 9

X. ◯ <u>14</u>, △ <u>13</u>, ☐ <u>10</u>

I. 41, 6, 39, 9, 21

VI.

goat	**peak**	**boil**	**half**
boat	*leak*	*coil*	*hale*
bolt	*lead*	*cool*	*bale*
colt	**head**	**cook**	**bake**

VII. 1) a,c,d   2) b,c   3) a,b,e   4) a,e   5) a,b,e

VIII.

99730	80692	126955	129957	108736
55509	111139	144366	145031	142599

IX. EXCISE, CERES, CRIES, EERIE, EXECS, RICES, SCREE, CERE, EXEC, ICES, IRES, RICE, RISE, SEER, SERE, SIRE,

X. $ 18 , % 12 , & 7

I.

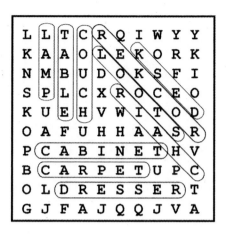

VI. a) 2:24am   b) 3:23pm or 15:23   c) 11:57am

VII. 1) a,c,d   2) b,c   3) a,b,e   4) a,e   5) c,d

VIII.   108990   99236   147788   119082   77113
         176349   64161   70935   132011   192017

IX. PUREE, RUPEE, EURO, PEER, PORE, POUR, PURE, ROPE,
    ROUE, ERE, ORE, OUR, ROE, RUE

X. All would live long, but none would be old.

I.

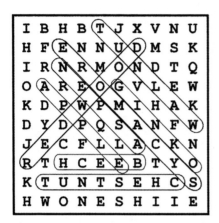

VI.

slick	**clock**	**date**
slice	*clack*	*rate*
spice	*slack*	*rats*
space	**snack**	*pats*
		pits

VII. My one regret in life is that I am not someone else.

VIII. a) 4:57pm or 16:57   b) 5:48pm or 17:48   c) 3:30pm or 15:30

IX. 23, 73, 8, 1, 57

X.   △ 9, □ 10, ◇ 11

I. 14, 14, 64, 14, 33

VI.

talk	**bill**	**rise**
tall	*ball*	*rile*
tell	*hall*	*file*
yell	**half**	*fill*
		fall

VII. 1) a,c,d   2) b,c   3) a,b,e   4) a,e   5) a,b,e

VIII.   78594   166551   163853   111368   85791
          113567   137575   100269   50980   124663

IX. FITFUL, CLIFF, FLUID, LICIT, LUCID, CUFF, CULT, DUCT,
    DUFF, FLIC, FLIT, LIFT, TIFF, TUFF

X.   △ 11,   □ 12, ▽ 10

I.

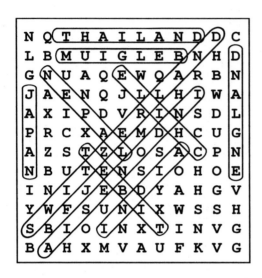

VI. a) 9:51pm or 21:51   b) 12:51am or 0:51   c) 4:39pm or 16:39

VII. 1) b,e   2) b,c   3) a,b,e   4) a,e   5) a,b,e

VIII.   106987   101823   86596   121325   107314
           114370   98472   112597   74968   116234

IX. VARLET, ALERT, ALTER, AVERT, LATER, RAVEL, VALET,
    EARL, LATE, LEAR, RATE, RAVE, REAL, TALE, TARE, TEAL,
    TEAR, VALE, VEAL

X. Nowadays men lead lives of noisy desperation.

I.

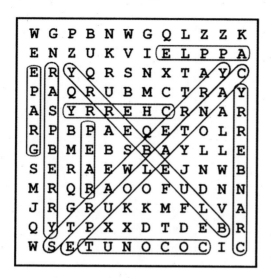

VI.

start	scone	slope	flag
stare	stone	scope	flap
store	stole	score	slap
stone	stale	scare	soap
			soar

VII. Repetition does not transform a lie into a truth.

VIII. a) 4 hours 58 min.   b) 222   c) 10:03am

IX. 14, 7, 243, -15, 96

X.   ∧ 12, < 11, > 7

I. 2, 3, 683, 11, 486

VI.

find	**calf**	**blow**	**sold**
bind	*call*	*blot*	*told*
band	*ball*	*boot*	*toll*
land	**bawl**	**boat**	*till*
			bill

VII. 1) a,c   2) a,b   3) a   4) b,c   5) a,c,e

VIII.

81785	85545	69500	58252	105105
98409	75650	157890	86583	25461

IX. CAMERA, CREAM, CRIME, ACRE, AREA, ARIA, CAME, CARE, CRAM, EMIR, MACE, MICA, MICE, MIRE, RACE, REAM, RICE

X. ☜ <u>11</u>, ☞ <u>10</u>, ☝ <u>17</u>

I.

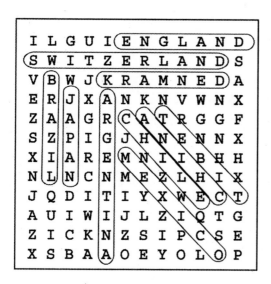

VI. a) 8 hours 55 min.   b) 21:25 or 9:25pm

VII. 1) a,b,e   2) b,c,e   3) a,d,e   4) a,c,d   5) a,d,e

VIII.   174538   103276   166357   135256   96613
            28827   17838   8603   36541   56757

IX. LOUPE, FLOP, FLUE, FOUL, FUEL, HELP, HOLE, HOPE,
    LOPE, POLE

X. California is a fine place to live, if you happen to be an orange.

Day 12   Solutions to Exercises

I.

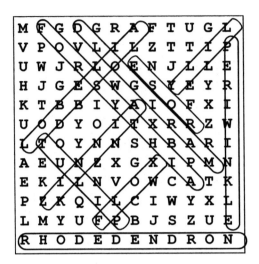

VI.

blow	snip	coal	trade
flow	*slip*	*goal*	*grade*
flaw	*flip*	*goad*	*glade*
flag	flap	gold	*blade*
			blame

VII. Silence is golden when you can't think of a good answer.

VIII. a) 16 hours 30 min.   b) 8 hours 10 min.   c) 1:00am or 01:00

IX. 3, 24, 2341, 4, 63

X.   ☺ <u>12</u>, ☺ <u>10</u>, ☹ <u>8</u>

I. 720, 222, 531246, 43, 481

VI.

yell	**head**	**toll**	**frog**
well	*hear*	*told*	*flog*
wall	*heir*	*toad*	*flop*
call	**hair**	**road**	*flip*
			slip
			skip

VII. 1) b,c,e   2) a,d   3) b,e   4) a,b   5) b,c,e

VIII.
99730	80692	126955	129957	108736
10254	1910	8934	5385	31039

IX. GATHER, HALTER, HAULER, HURTLE, LATHER, ALERT, ALTER, ARGUE, AUGER, AUGHT, EARTH, GLARE, GLUER, GRATE, GREAT, GRUEL, HATER, HAUTE, HEART, HUGER, LAGER, LARGE, LATER, LATHE, LAUGH, REGAL, RETAG, ULTRA

X.   ↗ 9, ↙ 10, ↘ 9

I.

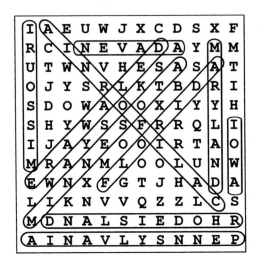

VI. a) 8:30am   b) 8 hours 10 min.   c) 9:30pm or 21:30

VII. 1) a,b,e   2) b,c   3) a,c,e   4) a,c,d   5) b,c,d

VIII.	55509	111139	144366	145031	142599
	9067	4873	41175	69877	10904

IX. FORMATION, INFORMANT, NOMINATOR, FOOTMAN,
    MARTINI, MONITOR, NONFARM, ORATION, ANOINT,
    FORMAT, INFANT, INFIRM, INFORM, MAROON, MARTIN,
    MATRON, MINION, MOTION, NATION, NONART, NONFAT,
    NOTION, RATION, TINMAN

X. When you get to the end of your rope, tie a knot and hang on.

I.

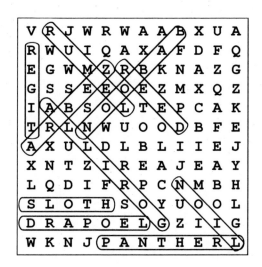

VI.

game	bawl	heat	bald
gate	ball	head	ball
gale	bell	held	hall
tale	yell	hold	hail
		cold	hair

VII. Age is a question of mind over matter. If you don't mind, it doesn't matter.

VIII. a) 6:00am   b) 11 hours 30 min.   c) 2:30am

IX. 4, 76, 642135, 2, 39

X.   △ 10,   ▽ 5,   ◁ 7,   ▷ 13

I. 19, 15, 7654, 33, 93

VI.

sport	**stow**
spore	*slow*
spare	*slot*
stare	*blot*
stars	*boot*
	boat

VII. 1) a,c   2) a,b,c   3) a,b,e   4) a,b,e   5) a,d

VIII. | 118146 | 184976 | 59833 | 125261 | 107168 |
|---|---|---|---|---|
| 18249 | 23997 | 2437 | 24564 | 29133 |

IX. SHINES, ENNUI, ISSUE, NINES, SHIES, SHINE, SHINS,
SHUNS, SINES, SINUS, SUSHI, HENS, HISS, HUES, HUNS,
INNS, NESS, NINE, NUNS, SHIN, SHUN, SINE, SINS, SUES,
SUNS, USES

X.   ☺ 12, ☺ 10, ☺ 9, ☺ 12

I.

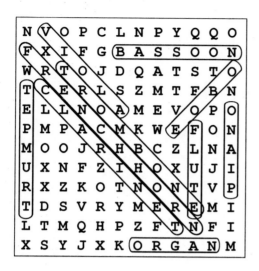

VI. a) 9:02am   b) 13 hours 25 min.   c) 3:05am

VII. 1) b,d,e   2) a,d   3) a,d   4) a,d,e   5) a,e

VIII.   82662   24165   122353   147539   84003
             19802   16551   14740   5630   19573

IX. ELATES, ESTATE, LATEST, LATTES, SETTLE, TEASEL,
    TESTAE, EASEL, ELATE, LATTE, LEASE, LEAST, SLATE,
    SLEET, STALE, STATE, STEAL, STEEL, TALES, TASTE, TEALS,
    TEASE

X. When the eagles are silent, the parrots begin to jabber.

I.

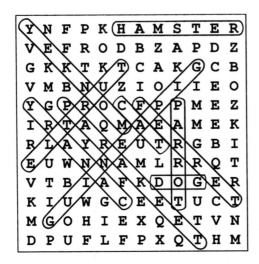

VI.

plant	**loot**
slant	boot
scant	boat
scans	goat
scars	goad
stars	**gold**

VII. It is better to know some of the questions than all of the answers.

VIII. a) 7:50am   b) 28 hours 5 min.   c) 11:55am

IX. 45, C, 26, M, 95

X. 🧍 <u>12</u>, 🙆 <u>7</u>, 🙋 <u>11</u>, 🙋 <u>9</u>

I. 46, 25, 66, S, 13

VI.

snow	blow
slow	blot
slot	boot
soot	bolt
coot	colt
coat	cold

VII. 1) a,d,e   2) a,d   3) a,b,d,e   4) d,e   5) a,b,d

VIII.   121257   173061   66618   94553   133912
           7030   4438   31312   30644   36914

IX. PRALINE, AERIAL, ALPINE, LINEAR, NAILER, PANIER,
PINEAL, PIRANA, PLANAR, PLANER, RAPINE, RENAIL,
REPLAN, ALIEN, APIAN, APNEA, ARENA, LEARN, LINER,
PAEAN, PALER, PANEL, PEARL, PENAL, PERIL, PLAIN,
PLANE, PLIER, RENAL, RIPEN

X.   12,   15,   9, 7

I.

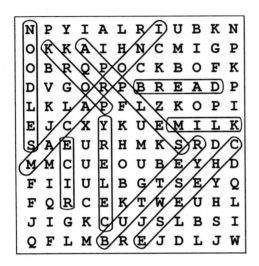

VI. a) 22 hours 30 min.   b) 11:43am   c) 5:41am

VII. 1) a,d   2) a,c,e   3) a,c,e   4) a,b,d,e   5) d,e

VIII.   139398   165640   143241   137924   144954
          21471   29993   11137   5084   11152

IX. BABELS, BALERS, BLARES, BRACES, CABLES, CLEARS,
    LACERS, RABBLE, SCALER, SCLERA, ABLER, ABLES, ACERB,
    ACRES, BABEL, BABES, BALER, BALES, BARBS, BARES,
    BASER, BEARS, BLABS, BLARE, BLASE, BLEAR, BRACE,
    CABLE, CARBS, CARES, CLEAR, CRABS, EARLS, LACER,
    LACES, LASER, LEARS, RACES, SABER, SABLE, SABRE, SCALE,
    SCARE

X. The future will be better tomorrow.

I.

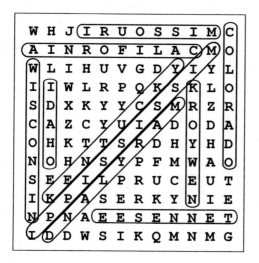

VI.

shun	**bait**
shin	*bail*
shim	*ball*
slim	*mall*
slum	*male*
slug	*mile*
	mice

VII. There's nothing worse than being an aging young person.

VIII. a) 9 hours 35 min.   b) 08:30am

IX. 32, R, FU, A, 47174

X.   ⌐↵ 13, ⌐→ 9, ↰→| 10, ↓↑ 8

I. 64, P, 67/13, 20, Q

VI.

hill	**slick**
till	*slice*
toll	*spice*
told	*spite*
toad	*spate*
road	**skate**

VII. 1) a,b,e 2) c,e 3) a,c,d 4) b,c,e 5) a,b,e

VIII.

52899	33575	37157	82383	151279
80791	17663	60774	4127	19604

IX. LARIATS, RITUALS, ALTARS, ASTRAL, LARIAT, RITUAL, TRAILS, TRIALS, ALIAS, ALTAR, ARIAS, ASTIR, ATLAS, AURAL, AURAS, LAIRS, LIARS, LIRAS, RAILS, SITAR, STAIR, SUTRA, TAILS, TIARA, TRAIL, TRIAL, ULTRA

X. ⤸ 7, ⤹ 13, ⤷ 9, ⤺ 4

I.

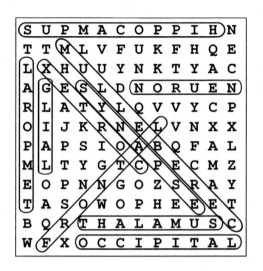

VI. a) 21 hours 7 min.   b) 5 hours 50 min.

VII. 1) a,c,e   2) b,e   3) a,c,e   4) a,d   5) c,d,e

VIII.   123545   53829   73410   137891   55668
              17979   40665   10011   16870   37349

IX. AEROBIC, ASCRIBE, BRAISE, CARIES, CAROBS, COARSE,
    COBRAS, ISOBAR, RABIES, SCRIBE, ACRES, ARISE, AROSE,
    BARES, BASIC, BEARS, BOARS, BORES, BORIC, BRACE,
    CARBS, CARES, CAROB, COBRA, CORES, CRABS, CRIBS,
    CRIES, ORCAS, RACES, RAISE, RICES, ROBES, SABER, SCARE,
    SCORE, SOBER

X. A fanatic is one who can't change his mind and won't change the
   subject.

I.

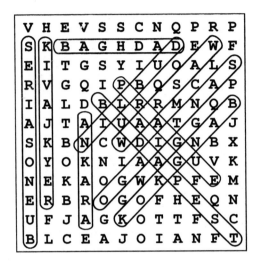

VI.

hand	**salt**
band	*sale*
bond	*sole*
fond	*sold*
food	*fold*
foot	**food**

VII. A problem cannot be solved by the same thinking that created it.

VIII. a) 4:11pm or 16:11   b) 5 hours 15 min.   c) 18 hours 10 min.

IX. 37, FV, 14, QP, H

X. 10, 7, 12, 7

I. 46, VE, 971, U, J

VI.

past	**lose**
vast	*lost*
vase	*most*
vise	*mist*
vine	*mint*
tine	*mind*
time	**find**

VII. 1) a,b,e   2) c,d   3) a,b,c   4) a,e   5) a,b,d

VIII.   161903   85576   105283   105829   145984
          14508   17048   15196   5528   12608

IX. NOVELTIES, INVITEES, NOVELIST, EVILEST, INVITEE,
    INVITES, LIONISE, SETLINE, SOLVENT, TENSILE, VIOLENT,
    VIOLETS, VIOLINS, VIOLIST, ELITES, ENLIST, ENVIES,
    EVENTS, INLETS, INSOLE, INSTIL, VIOLET, VIOLIN, INVITE

X. 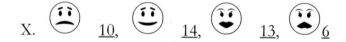 10,   14,   13,   6

I.

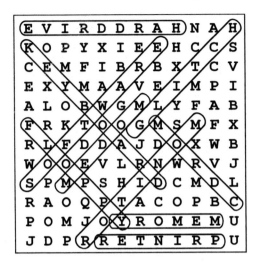

VI. a) 3 hours 45 min. b) 8 hours 50 min. c) 11:15pm or 23:15

VII. 1) c,d,e 2) a,b,d,e 3) a,c,e 4) a,b,d 5) a,b,e

VIII.

30804	77481	63234	118526	82082
66219	28397	28107	23572	26112

IX. CLEATS, CASTE, CELTS, CLEAT, ECLAT, LACES, LEAST, SCALE, SLATE, STALE, STEAL, TALCS, TALES, TEALS, ACES, ACTS, ALES, CASE, CAST, CATS, CELT, EAST, EATS, LACE, LAST, LATE, LEST, LETS, SALE, SALT, SATE, SCAT, SEAL, SEAT, SECT, SLAT, TALC, TALE, TEAL

X. Eighty percent of success is showing up.

I.

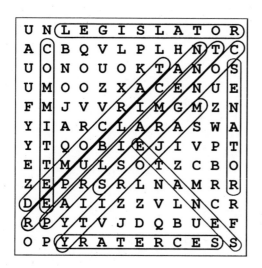

VI.

kiss	slow
miss	slot
mils	soot
mild	moot
mold	most
told	mast
toad	fast

VII. It is easier to stay out than to get out.

VIII. a) 9:22am   b) 24 hours 13 min.   c) 5 hours 15 min.

IX. 472, WH, 96, FL, JK

X. ॐ 12, ॐ 9, ॐ 11, ॐ 7

I. 487, TH, GBH, KKL, HF

VI.

take	book
tale	*rook*
tall	*rock*
tail	*rack*
fail	*race*
foil	*rage*
fool	**page**

VII. 1) b,d,e   2) a,b,e   3) c,d,e   4) a,c,e   5) a,c,d

VIII.

75579	120902	134633	137361	57451
11075	46966	17504	33747	71164

IX. CLIENTELE, TELEGENIC, ELECTING, ENTICING
LENIENCE, CEILING, GENETIC, GENTEEL, GENTILE,
GILLNET, INCLINE, LENIENT, LIGNITE, LILTING,
NEGLECT, TELLING, TILLING, CITING, CLIENT, ELICIT,
ENGINE, ENTICE, GENTLE, IGNITE, INCITE, LENTEN,
LENTIL, LIGNIN, LINING, LINNET, LINTEL,
TEEING, TILING, TINGLE, TINING

X.　 <u>10,</u>　 <u>9,</u>　 <u>10,</u>　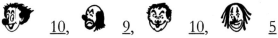 <u>5</u>